The role of antihormones

Current controversies in the
treatment of breast cancer

Volume 1

The role of antihormones

Edited by A Howell

The Parthenon Publishing Group
International Publishers in Science, Technology & Education

Casterton Hall, Carnforth,
Lancs. LA6 2LA, UK

120 Mill Road, Park Ridge,
New Jersey 07656, USA

Published in the UK by
The Parthenon Publishing Group Limited
Casterton Hall, Carnforth,
Lancs, LA6 2LA, England

Published in the USA by
The Parthenon Publishing Group Inc.
120 Mill Road,
Park Ridge,
New Jersey 07656, USA

British Library Cataloguing-in-Publication Data
The role of antihormones.
  1. Women. Breasts. Cancer. Therapy
  I. Howell, A.   II. Series
  616.9944906

  ISBN 1-85070-295-0

Library of Congress Cataloging-in-Publication Data
The Role of antihormones / edited by A. Howell.
        p.   cm. – (Current controversies in the treatment of breast
  cancer : v. 1)
      Includes bibliographical references.
      Includes index.
      ISBN 1-85070-295-0
  1. Breast – Cancer – Chemotherapy. 2. Hormone antagonists – Therapeutic
  use. 3. Breast – Cancer – Hormone therapy.   I. Howell,
  A. (Anthony)   II. Series.
      [DNLM: 1. Breast Neoplasms – drug therapy. 2. Buserelin Acetate –
  analogs & derivatives. 3. Hormone Antagonists – therapeutic use.
  WP 870 R7448]
  RC280.B8RS   1990
  616.99'449061 – dc20
  DNLM/DLC
  for Library of Congress   90-14177
                                                                   CIP

First published 1991

Composition by Ryburn Typesetting Ltd, Halifax, England
Printed and bound in Great Britain by
Butler and Tanner, Frome and London

Contents

List of principal contributors

R.W. Blamey
City Hospital
Hucknall Road
Nottingham NG5 1PB
UK

W. Eiermann
Department of Gynaecology and
   Obstetrics
Klinikum Grosshadern
Ludwig-Maximilians Universität
Marchioninistrasse 15
D-8000 Munich 70
Munich
West Germany

B.J.A. Furr
ICI Pharmaceuticals
Alderley Park
Macclesfield
Cheshire SK10 4TF
UK

A. Howell
Department of Medical Oncology
Christie Hospital and Holt Radium
   Institute
Wilmslow Road
Manchester M20 9BX
UK

M. Kaufmann
Department of Obstetrics and
   Gynaecology
University Hospital
D-6900 Heidelberg
West Germany

J.G.M. Klijn
Division of Endocrine Oncology
Rotterdam Cancer Institute
Dr Daniel den Hoed Cancer Center
Groene Hilledijk 301
P.O. Box 5201
3008 AE Rotterdam
The Netherlands

J. Lewis
ICI Pharmaceuticals
Alderley Park
Macclesfield
Cheshire SK10 4TF
UK

R. Mansel
University Hospital of South
   Manchester
Nell Lane
West Didsbury
Manchester M20 8LR
UK

R.I. Nicholson
Breast Cancer Unit
Tenovus Institute for Cancer
  Research
University of Wales College of
  Medicine
Heath Park
Cardiff CF4 4XX
UK

Y. Nomura
Department of Breast Surgery
National Kyushu Cancer Centre
Fukuoka
Japan

R. Peto
Clinical Trial Service Unit 6
  ICRF Cancer Studies Unit
Radcliffe Infirmary
Oxford OX2 6HE
UK

P.E. Preece
University Department of Surgery
Ninewells Hospital and Medical
  School
Dundee DD1 9SY
UK

C. Rose
Department of Oncology R
Odense University Hospital
DK-5000 Odense C
Denmark

A.E. Wakeling
ICI Pharmaceuticals
Alderley Park
Macclesfield
Cheshire SK10 4TF
UK

Section I

Management of premenopausal advanced breast cancer

1

Systemic therapy of metastatic breast cancer

C. Rose

INTRODUCTION

The primary goal in the treatment of patients with metastatic breast cancer is to achieve maximal palliation of the symptoms with minimal toxicity and with the longest possible time to progression. Since optimal efficacy of cytotoxic therapy had been reached during the 1970s by achieving response rates of 60% and median times to progression of 8–12 months, the various endocrine therapies have attracted renewed interest used alone, in combination with each other, or in addition to cytotoxic therapy. The efficacy and low toxicity of the antioestrogen tamoxifen has been established in comparative trials with other ablative, additive, or inhibitive treatment approaches[1]. Although none of these trials have included a large enough number of patients to allow detection of even quite large differences in response rate (10–20%), these trials have been of prime importance in placing tamoxifen as the treatment of choice for first-line endocrine therapy. Furthermore, a number of trials have explored the possibility of an increased efficacy by combining tamoxifen with other endocrine approaches. Since the mode of action and toxicities for cytotoxic and endocrine therapies are different, and since experimental, pathological, and clinical data substantiate the concept that breast carcinomas are heterogeneous, it is attractive to explore new approaches by combining cytotoxic and endocrine treatment of

3

metastatic breast cancer in order to prolong survival[2].

In the following, a short summary of data from trials of tamoxifen, and other endocrine therapies will be given. Secondly, data will be presented from trials of combined endocrine therapy where tamoxifen is used as one of the endocrine modalities. Finally, the results from trials analysing cytotoxic therapy and tamoxifen given in combination will be summarized.

All the data given are based upon previously published reviews[1,2] and the reader is referred to these reviews for the relevant references.

ENDOCRINE THERAPY OF METASTATIC BREAST CANCER

Tamoxifen has been compared with other endocrine modalities in 26 randomized trials, which are summarized in Table 1. A rate of response in the order of 30–35% has been found, regardless of whether treatment has been by tamoxifen, oophorectomy, aminoglutethimide and hydrocortisone, oestrogens, medroxyprogesterone acetate, or megestrole acetate. In the trials analysing the efficacy of androgens versus tamoxifen there is a trend towards a lower response rate for patients treated with androgens as first-line endocrine therapy.

By analysing the cross-over data given in some of the trials summarized in Table 1, it appears from Tables 2 and 3 that the response rate to a

Table 1 Response (%) to tamoxifen compared to other endocrine modalities in advanced breast cancer. Summary of 26 randomized trials

No. of trials	Tamoxifen		Comparative therapy		
	n	*(%)*	*n*	*(%)*	
2	81	(25)	79	(27)	ovariectomy
1	26	(35)	25	(52)	adrenalectomy
6	248	(27)	249	(28)	oestrogens
3	123	(26)	136	(18)	androgens
12	696	(34)	762	(35)	progestins
2	99	(33)	93	(32)	aminoglutethimide + hydrocortisone

Table 2 Cross-sensitivity (%) between tamoxifen (TAM) and other endocrine therapies (ET)

No. of trials	Response to TAM in responders to comparative ET		Response to comparative ET in responders to TAM		
	n	*(%)*	*n*	*(%)*	
1	7	(14)	5	(40)	ovariectomy
1	6	(17)	2	(50)	adrenalectomy
4	11	(36)	22	(36)	oestrogens
5	15	(13)	7	(33)	progestins
3	20	(25)	26	(39)	aminoglutethimide + hydrocortisone

Table 3 Non-cross-resistance (%) between tamoxifen (TAM) and other endocrine therapies (ET)

No. of trials	Response to TAM in non-responders to comparative ET		Response to comparative ET in non-responders to TAM		
	n	*(%)*	*n*	*(%)*	
1	11	(9)	10	(30)	ovariectomy
1	9	(22)	7	(57)	adrenalectomy
4	52	(21)	41	(17)	oestrogens
1	20	(15)	10	(10)	oestrogens
5	53	(6)	104	(10)	progestins
3	42	(7)	61	(12)	aminoglutethimide + hydrocortisone

second-line treatment by tamoxifen in patients who have responded to a previous endocrine treatment is lower than the response rate to any other second-line endocrine therapy in patients who have first responded to tamoxifen. For patients who have not responded to first-line endocrine therapy, the response rate to second-line therapy is essentially independent of treatment modality and is approximately 10% (Table 3). However, the response rate tends to be higher when tamoxifen is given as the first therapy. Since the toxicity profiles from the various endocrine therapies are so different, a direct comparison seems almost meaningless. However, in comparison with other endocrine modality treatments, tamoxifen is generally without major side-effects.

EVALUATION OF THE POSSIBLE CANDIDATES FOR ENDOCRINE THERAPY IN PRE- AND POSTMENOPAUSAL METASTATIC BREAST CANCER

Premenopausal metastatic breast cancer

Castration, either by surgery or by irradiation, is the oldest form of endocrine therapy, and until recently it was considered to be the treatment of choice in all premenopausal patients with metastatic disease. The overall response rate in 1674 premenopausal patients has been found to be 33%. Surgical and radiation castration have never been compared in a randomized trial but they have produced similar response rates. It is therefore reasonable to suggest that ovarian ablation by radiotherapy can substitute for surgical procedures because of its lower cost. Very high doses of oestrogens have been tried in premenopausal patients and seem to be without effect. Androgens can be used to induce menostasia, but this requires high doses that lead to unacceptable virilization. In the only two randomized comparisons between tamoxifen and oophorectomy (Table 4), although the numbers are small, similar rates of response are obtained and there is no difference in median length of survival.

Postmenopausal metastatic breast cancer

Because of the relative cheapness of treatment with oestrogens, the randomized comparisons between tamoxifen and diethylstiboestrol or ethinyloestradiol have been summarized (Table 5). The various treatment end-points are comparable between the two treatment options and without significant differences. Although the side-effects of oestrogen treatment are claimed to be less severe with continued treatment, all six

Table 4 Randomized trials comparing tamoxifen (TAM) with oophorectomy in metastatic breast cancer

References	Treatment (daily dose)	Response rate CR+PR/n*	%	Response duration (days, median)	Time to treatment failure (days, median)	Survival (days, median)
Ingle *et al.*	TAM (20 mg)	7/26	27	453	160	749
	ovariectomy	10/27	37	476	144	722
Buchanan *et al.*	TAM (40 mg)	13/55	24	600	—	450
	ovariectomy	11/52	21	210	—	750

*CR, complete remission; PR, partial remission

Table 5 Randomized trials comparing tamoxifen and oestrogens in metastatic breast cancer

References	Treatment* (daily dose)	Response rate CR+PR/n	%	Response duration (days, median)	Time to treatment failure (days, median)	Survival (days, median)
Stewart et al.	TAM (10 mg x 3)	9/29	31	266	—	—
	DES (5 mg x 3)	6/27	22	228	—	—
Ingle et al.	TAM (10 mg x 2)	23/69	33	238	171	735
	DES (5 mg x 3)	30/74	41	393	142	>1140
Ribeiro	TAM (20 mg)	13/47	28	720	—	—
	DES (3 mg)	14/45	31	720	—	—
Gockerman et al.	TAM (10 mg x 2)	3/54	6	—	150	1020
	DES (5 mg x 3)	5/50	10	—	180	1050
Beex et al.	TAM (20 mg x 2)	10/30	33	330	—	750
	EE$_2$ (3 mg)	9/29	31	360	—	930
Matelski et al.	TAM (20 mg)	10/10	53	—	—	—
	EE$_2$ (3 mg)	6/24	25	—	—	—

*TAM, tamoxifen; DES, diethylstilboestrol; EE$_2$, ethinyloestradiol

randomized trials clearly show that the toxicity of tamoxifen is less. Oestrogen treatment had to be discontinued due to side-effects in about 50% of patients in two of the trials. Even in the study by Ribeiro, using only 3 mg of diethylstiboestrol daily, 15% of the patients had to stop treatment. In spite of the substantial proportion of patients stopping treatment because of side-effects, this did not seem to influence the results of treatment with oestrogens.

Based upon the relative efficacy of the various endocrine treatment modalities and their toxicity, it seems justified to conclude that first choice of the endocrine therapy in both pre- and postmenopausal women is tamoxifen.

COMBINED ENDOCRINE THERAPY

The clinical finding of partial cross-sensitivity and a lack of complete cross-resistance between the different endocrine treatments indicates that these therapies may not share the same mode of action. Thus there is a rationale for the simultaneous combination of different endocrine therapies. Many investigators have explored the effect of combined endocrine therapy in randomized trials. The results from trials of tamoxifen in combination with either androgens, aminoglutethimide and hydrocortisone, or glucocorticoids in metastatic breast cancer are shown in Tables 6 and 7. In four out of five trials analysing the addition of androgen to tamoxifen, a trend towards an increased response rate is demonstrated. Preliminary data from the largest of these trials (Wallgren *et al.*) even suggest a survival advantage for the combined approach. The addition of aminoglutethimide, hydrocortisone and danazol to tamoxifen led to an increase in response rate. This was not, however, translated into a prolongation of survival. In the two consecutive trials an increased response rate has been obtained by combining prednisolone and tamoxifen. In the second of these trials, a preliminary analysis indicates that the higher rate of response was followed by a prolongation of survival.

Although some of these results seem promising, there is no strong evidence at the present time for combining endocrine therapies in routine practice. However, the addition of prednisolone to tamoxifen merits further study.

Table 6 Randomized trials of tamoxifen in combination with androgens in metastatic breast cancer

References	Treatment* (daily dose)	Response rate CR+PR/n	%	Response duration (days, median)	Time to treatment failure (days, median)	Survival (days, median)
Thomey et al.	TAM (2–100 mg/m² x 2)	8/52	15	230	64	330
	TAM (2–100 mg/m² x 2)	21/56	37	212	180	380
	FLU (7 mg/m² x 2)					
Twito et al.	TAM (10 mg x 2)	50/119	42	—	199	860
	TAM (10 mg x 2)	62/120	52	—	364	917
	FLU (10 mg x 2)					
Rose et al.	TAM (10 mg x 3)	32/94	34	720	300	720
	TAM (10 mg x 3)	36/87	44	720	330	720
	FLU (5 mg x 4)					
Wallgren et al.	TAM (20 mg x 2)	36/145	25	615	—	964
	TAM (20 mg x 2)	51/139	37	>720	—	696
	FLU (10 mg x 2)					
Heinonen et al.	TAM (10 mg x 3)	24/49	49	—	>390	870
	TAM (10 mg x 3)	22/49	45	—	>360	750
	NAND (100 mg i.m/w/2.w.)					

*TAM, tamoxifen; FLU, fluoxymesterone; NAND, nandrolone

Table 7 Randomized trials of tamoxifen in combination with inhibitive endocrine therapy of glucocorticoids in metastatic breast cancer

References	Treatment* (daily dose)	Response rate CR+PR/n	%	Response duration (days, median)	Time to treatment failure (days, median)	Survival (days, median)
Powles et al.	TAM (10 mg x 2)	34/111	31	675	—	1440 (CR+PR)
	TAM (10 mg x 2) AG+H (250 mg x 2 + 20 mg x 2) Danazol (100 mg x 3)	48/111	43	540	—	690 (CR+PR)
Milsted et al.	TAM (10 mg x 2)	5/26	19	—	—	—
	TAM (10 mg x 2) AG+H (250 mg x 4 + 10 mg x 2)	6/26	23	—	—	—
Ingle et al.	TAM (10 mg x 2)	21/49	43	452	216	657
	TAM (10 mg x 2) AG+H (250 mg x 4 + 100 mg x 4)	25/51	49	447	227	827
Rose et al.	TAM (10 mg x 3)	32/94	34	720	300	720
	TAM (10 mg x 3) AG+H (250 mg x 4 + 20 mg x 3)	24/83	29	720	240	720
Stewart et al.	TAM (10 mg x 2)	9/72	13	390	—	360
	TAM (10 mg x 2) Pred. (5 mg x 2)	26/73	36	390	—	630
Rubens et al.†	TAM (10 mg x 2)	24/77	31	360	—	NS‡
	TAM (10 mg x 2) Pred. (5 mg x 2)	39/85	46	720	—	NS

*TAM, tamoxifen; AG+H, aminoglutethimide + hydrocortisone; pred, prednisolone; †Personal communication; ‡NS, not significant

COMBINED CYTOTOXIC AND ENDOCRINE THERAPY

Cytotoxic therapy has been combined with ablative, additive, or competitive treatment modalities. Furthermore, the combination of cytotoxic and endocrine therapies has been applied either simultaneously, sequentially, or alternately. Tables 8 and 9 summarize the data from trials where tamoxifen has been given in combination with cytotoxic therapy either simultaneously or sequentially. The trials by Cavalli and co-workers and the Australian/New Zealand Breast Cancer Group demonstrate that tamoxifen therapy followed by cytotoxic therapy upon progression is as effective in terms of overall response rate and survival as cytotoxic treatment and tamoxifen given simultaneously in postmenopausal patients with metastatic breast cancer.

Although the biological rationale for the combined therapy of cytotoxic drugs and tamoxifen appears sound in theory, at present there is no reason for combining these modalities as a routine in patients with metastatic breast cancer.

Table 8 Simultaneous cytotoxic and endocrine therapy

References	Therapy*	n	%	Survival
Cocconi	CMF	71	51	777
	CMF+TAM	62	74	546
CMEA	CMF	82	40	—
	CMF+TAM	71	41	—
Mouridsen	CMF	105	49	570
	CMF+TAM	115	75	720
Krook	CFP	65	68	544
	CFP+TAM	59	61	394
Viladiu	CMF	33	46	675
	CMF+TAM	34	71	741
	CMF+MPA	31	68	651

*CMF, cyclophosphamide + methotrexate + 5-fluorouracil; TAM, tamoxifen; CFP, cyclophosphamide + 5-fluorouracil + prednisone; MPA, medroxypro-gesterone acetate

Table 9 Sequential cytotoxic and endocrine therapy

Reference	1 Line	n	%	2 Line	n	%	Survival
Glick	TAM*	88	49	TAM	33	85	—
				TAM+CMF	29	87	—
				CMF	—	—	—
Bezwoda	TAM	24	63	CMF	9	33	513
	TAM+CMF	26	65	—	—	—	531
Cocconi	CMF	71	51	CMF+TAM	39	31	777
	CMF+TAM	62	74	—	—	—	546
Cavalli	TAM	145	17	CT	145	16	825
	TAM+CT	152	40	—	—	—	711
AUST.N-Z.	TAM	113	22	AC	72	35	630
	TAM+AC	113	51	—	—	—	600
	AC	113	45	TAM	55	6	540

*TAM, tamoxifen; CMF, cyclophosphamide + methotrexate + 5-fluorouracil; AC, adriamycin + cyclophosphamide; CT, cytotoxic therapy

CONCLUSION

Considering efficacy and side-effects of the various options for endocrine therapy, and assuming that every patient with metastatic disease should have at least one trial of endocrine therapy, one can justifiably conclude that tamoxifen seems to be the treatment of choice for first-line endocrine therapy in both pre- and postmenopausal breast cancer patients.

Despite an obvious clinical rationale for combined endocrine therapy most trials have failed to show any benefit. Although data from trials combining tamoxifen with prednisolone or an androgen seem promising, the use of combined endocrine therapy cannot at present be recommended outside the context of randomized clinical trials. By combining tamoxifen and cytotoxic therapy most trials demonstrate an increase in response rate in the order of what can be expected on the basis of an assumption of independent biological actions of the two treatment modalities. In spite of the increase of rate of response, no prolongation of survival has been observed. The combined cytotoxic–endocrine approach is therefore a field which deserves further investigation.

REFERENCES

1. Rose, C. and Mouridsen, H. T. (1988). Endocrine therapy of advanced breast cancer. *Acta Oncol.*, **27**, 721–8
2. Rose, C. and Mouridsen, H. T. (1984). Combined cytotoxic and endocrine therapy in breast cancer. In Bresciani, F. *et al.* (eds.) *Progress Cancer Research and Therapy*, vol. 31, pp. 269–86. (New York: Raven Press)

2

Review of the endocrine actions of LHRH agonists in premenopausal women with advanced breast cancer

R.I. Nicholson, K.J. Walker, J.F.R. Robertson and R.W. Blamey

INTRODUCTION

Our interest in luteinizing hormone releasing hormone (LHRH) analogues began in 1977 following an approach by ICI Pharmaceuticals division in the United Kingdom to screen a series of LHRH agonists which they believed might have interesting endocrinological and antitumour properties. The results obtained at that time clearly showed that in the mature female rat the secondary effects produced by the agonists were very much dependent upon the dose and duration of exposure to the drug. When they were administered at low levels as a single injection they were able to mimic the actions of LHRH, however, when given at high concentrations over prolonged periods of time they produced antireproductive effects[1]. Indeed, when ICI 118,630, now know clinically as Zoladex (D-Ser (Bu^t)^6, Azgly^{10}, LHRH; goserelin) was administered to mature female Sprague–Dawley rats at 5 μg twice daily for several weeks it rapidly reduced ovarian activity, decreased circulating concentrations of oestradiol and progesterone, with secondary hypoprolactinaemia, decreased the size of oestrogen target tissues, including the uterus and mammary gland[2-4] and caused extensive remissions in oestrogen receptor (ER)-positive, dimethylbenzanthracene-induced mammary tumours[2,3]. Significantly, many of these effects were recognized as being similar to those induced by surgical castration[1,5-7], an observation which forms the

15

basis for the use of LHRH agonists in the therapy of hormone-sensitive cancers of the breast and reproductive tract and their benign conditions[8-11].

Against this background, the current article reviews aspects of the endocrinological properties of LHRH agonists in advanced breast cancer patients. Although emphasis is placed on our own studies with Zoladex, where relevant, comparisons are made with results obtained using the LHRH agonists buserelin (D-Ser(Bu^t)^6, LHRH proethylamide[9]), leuprolide (D-Leu^6, LHRH proethylamide[9]) and decapeptyl (D-Trp^6, LHRH) and also with surgical and X-ray-induced castration in breast cancer patients. In adopting this approach it is envisaged that the strengths and limitations of LHRH agonist therapy will become apparent and aid in our assessment of their likely role in the modern management of diseases of the breast and reproductive tract.

ENDOCRINE ACTIONS OF LHRH AGONISTS IN PREMENOPAUSAL WOMEN WITH ADVANCED BREAST CANCER

The endocrine effects of either daily injections of Zoladex or a sustained-release formulation of the drug on circulating levels of ovarian and pituitary gland hormones have been reviewed elsewhere[7]. In the present communication these data will be summarized in an updated form.

The patterns of luteinizing hormone (LH) and follicle stimulating hormone (FSH) released during treatment with the LHRH agonist are quantitatively similar in individual patients and appear largely independent of whether treatment is initiated during the follicular or luteal phase of the menstrual cycle. Thus, elevated gonadotropins are observed in all patients after the first exposure to the drug and are followed by a subsequent reduction of their basal levels. The reduction occurs as a function of pituitary gland desensitization and has been maintained for periods of up to 2 years. Small rises in circulating oestradiol and progesterone are often associated with the early increased plasma concentrations of the gonadotropins. The levels obtained, however, are within the normal premenopausal range for these hormones. On continued treatment plasma oestradiol and progesterone concentrations decrease and fall to the castrate or postmenopausal range within 3 to 4 weeks. The ability of Zoladex to reduce circulating concentrations of oestradiol is not influenced by patient age (range, 34–50 years) or weight (range, 46–100 kg)[10]. Similarly, no relationship between these parameters and plasma levels of LH, FSH and progesterone has been found. Comparison of the published data on the ability of Zoladex[7,12], buserelin[13] and leuprolide[14] to reduce circulating levels of oestradiol and progesterone does not reveal any striking differences in the effectiveness of these drugs, each promotes a very significant decline in the level of these hormones within 1 month. Differences do, however, exist in the dose and mode of administration of the drugs, with the sustained-release depots providing the most convenient formulation. It is noteworthy that the rate of decline in the circulating concentrations of oestradiol and progesterone achieved by LHRH agonist therapy is not as rapid as that produced by the surgical removal of the ovaries, where the plasma levels of these hormones reach postmenopausal levels within 2 to 7 days[15,16].

Plasma levels of oestrone, androstenedione and testosterone are also reduced by LHRH agonist therapy[17,18]. The decreases are not as dramatic as those seen for oestradiol and progesterone and, although producing levels equivalent to those determined in postmenopausal women during Zoladex therapy[10], represent only a 10–30% fall in the circulating levels of these hormones. Finally, a reduction is also seen in the circulating level of prolactin in long-term Zoladex-treated patients[10], an observation in contrast to the lack of effect of buserelin[13] and leuprolide[18] on this hormone.

SIDE-EFFECTS OF LHRH AGONIST THERAPY

The side-effects relating to treatment with LHRH agonists are minimal and are primarily associated with the hypo-oestrogenic state. They include cessation of menstruation, hot flushes and occasional nausea[13,18,19]: effects common to surgical oophorectomy[20]. All suppressed patients have ceased to have normal menstrual periods by 2 months, although spotting has been recorded in one study using daily injections of Zoladex[7]. Local irritation can occur at the site of injection. Significantly, to date, increased pain soon after starting LHRH agonist therapy has only been reported in two of 120 patients and was not thought to be true tumour flare[18]. Comparison of ovarian histology in primary oophorectomized and Zoladex-treated premenopausal patients with advanced breast cancer has not revealed any gross abnormalities in the ovaries of long-term LHRH agonist-treated patients[21]. Indeed, no significant differences in the numbers of primordial, primary and secondary follicles have been observed between the two groups. There was, however, a significant reduction in the number of corpora lutea in Zoladex-treated patients. Interestingly, this corresponds to a slight increase in the number of follicular cysts, which may arise from atretic follicles which have previously failed to ovulate under the inhibitory actions of the drug. No abnormal pathology was ascribed to the cysts.

MECHANISM OF LHRH AGONIST ACTION

These endocrine data, although based on early clinical studies, indicate that the relatively quiescent state within the gonads of long-term LHRH agonist-treated patients most likely results from the ability of LHRH agonists to down-regulate pituitary LHRH receptors and hence desensitize the pituitary gland to the releasing-hormone properties of the drug[9]. This process eventually results in a fall in circulating levels of LH and FSH and a withdrawal of their support for gonadal steroidogenic activity. Since both primary and secondary follicles are seen in the ovaries of LHRH agonist-treated patients[21], it appears that an inhibition of ovarian steroidogenic processes can occur independently of early follicular development. These data are similar to those described in hypophysectomized rats, where follicular growth up to the size of the largest non-ovulatory follicles takes place in the complete absence of the gonadotropins and reduced ovarian steroid levels[22,23]. As folliculogenesis continues up to the point of ovulation while patients are on Zoladex, it may be expected that if therapy is stopped ovulation would recommence and the patient would again become fertile, an important consideration when LHRH agonists are to be used to treat benign diseases of the breast.

CONCLUSIONS AND FUTURE PROSPECTS

Clearly LHRH agonists represent an interesting addition to the spectrum of drugs currently available to treat hormone-sensitive breast cancer in premenopausal women. Their modest side-effects and ease of administration provide a contrast to the risks, trauma and morbidity of surgical endocrine therapy and represent clinically important considerations in light of:

(1)   The failure of all patients to respond to endocrine measures and their palliative nature;

(2)   Our inability in all centres to predict response and duration of remission;

(3)   The unsuitability of surgical oophorectomy in patients debilitated by their disease; and,

(4)   The unacceptability in some patients, of surgical and, therefore, irreversible procedures.

Indeed, Kardinal and Donegan[24] have stated that the risk of death following surgical castration in patients with advanced cancer is approximately 4% and results from the failure of vital organs extensively damaged by metastases. Similar rates of early postoperative deaths have been reported by Taylor[25], Fracchia *et al.*[26] and Lee and Hori[27]. Although LHRH agonist therapy should presumably avoid this mortality, a limiting feature of treatment with these drugs, as with X-ray induced menopause, may ultimately stem from their inability to suppress ovarian activity immediately (3 to 4 weeks) in patients with rapidly progressing disease and in patients with severe pain.

In addition to the use of LHRH agonists as single agents in premenopausal breast cancer patients, they are also being examined in combination with other endocrine therapies. Emphasis is initially being placed on their actions in combination with the antioestrogen tamoxifen, since although they share a common line of action through their involvement with oestrogens, nevertheless it is envisaged that they have non–overlapping mechanisms of action. The studies are, therefore, based on the rationale that while LHRH agonists reduce ovarian activity, they do not interfere with peripheral oestradiol production, a factor which is believed to play a major role in the promotion of hormone-sensitive breast cancer growth in postmenopausal women, and that the effects of this may be inhibited by the antioestrogen. Other arguments favouring combined therapies include the possibility that they might reduce the risk of early tumour flare and shorten the time required to achieve a full suppression of ovarian activity[18]. Significantly, our early endocrine studies in pre- and perimenopausal advanced breast cancer patients have not to date indicated any adverse interactions between the drugs, indeed the combination of Zoladex plus tamoxifen causes a fuller suppression of pituitary and ovarian function than Zoladex alone[28]. Moreover, in groups of women followed up for 1 year, the circulating concentrations of FSH and oestradiol are significantly lower in patients using the combination. The clinical efficacy of Zoladex plus tamoxifen versus Zoladex alone is currently under evaluation in a randomized multicentre trial (ICI study 2302). Patients who are initially randomized to receive Zoladex alone are given tamoxifen if they show objective progression while on treatment. Similarly, early studies examining the endocrinological actions of buserelin plus tamoxifen in premenopausal women, and which indicated no adverse interactions between the drugs when an adequate formulation of buserelin is used[29], are being clinically appraised in a European Organization for Research and Treatment of Cancer (EORTC) randomized study, as are combinations of leuprolide and tamoxifen[18].

ACKNOWLEDGEMENTS

The authors wish to thank the Tenovus Organization for their generous financial support.

REFERENCES

1. Maynard, P.V. and Nicholson, R.I. (1979). Biological effects of high dose levels of a series of new LH-RH analogues to intact female rats. *Br. J. Cancer*, **39**, 274–9
2. Nicholson, R.I. and Maynard, P.V. (1979). Antitumour activity of ICI 118630, a new potent luteinizing hormone-releasing hormone agonist. *Br. J. Cancer*, **39**, 268–73
3. Nicholson, R.I., Walker, K.J. and Maynard, P.V. (1980). Anti-tumour potential of a new luteinizing hormone-releasing hormone analogue ICI 118630. In Mouridsen, H.T. and Palshof, T. (eds.) *Breast Cancer, Experimental and Clinical Aspects*, pp. 295–9. (Oxford: Pergamon Press)
4. Nicholson, R.I., Gotting, K.E., Gee, J. and Walker, K.J. (1988). Actions of oestrogens and antioestrogens on rat mammary gland development: relevance to breast cancer prevention. *J. Steroid Biochem.*, **30**, 95–103
5. Nicholson, R.I., Walker, K.J., Harper, M., Phillips, A.D. and Furr, B.J.A. (1983). Future use of luteinizing hormone-releasing hormone agonists in the therapy of breast cancer in pre- and post-menopausal women. In

Nicholson, R.I. and Griffiths, K. (eds.) *Reviews on Endocrine-Related Cancer: Breast Cancer*, Suppl. 13, pp. 52–62. (Macclesfield: ICI Publications)

6. Nicholson, R.I., Walker, K.J., Davies, P. *et al.* (1984). Use and mechanism of action of the LH-RH agonist ICI 118630 in the therapy of hormone sensitive breast and prostate cancer. In Bresciani, F., King, R.J.B. and Lippman, M.F. (eds.) *Hormones and Cancer 2: Proceedings of the International Congress on Hormones and Cancer*, pp. 519–32. (New York: Raven Press)

7. Nicholson, R.I., Walker, K.J. and Turkes, A. *et al.* (1984). Therapeutic significance and mechanism of action of the LH-RH agonist ICI 118630 in breast and prostate cancer. *J. Steroid Biochem.*, **20**, 129–35

8. Schally, A.V., Redding, T.W. and Comaru-Schally, A.V. (1984). Potential use of analogues of luteinizing hormone-releasing hormone in the treatment of hormone sensitive neoplasms. *Cancer Treat. Rep.*, **68**, 281–9

9. Nicholson, R.I. and Walker, K.J. (1988). Preclinical studies and antitumour mechanism of action of LH-RH analogues. In Osborne, C.K. (ed.) *Endocrine Therapies in Breast and Prostate Cancer*, pp. 1–23. (Boston: Kluwer Academic Publishers)

10. Nicholson, R.I. and Walker, K.J. (1989). Use of LH-RH agonists in the treatment of breast disease. *R. Soc. Edinburgh*, **95**, 271–82

11. Nicholson, R.I. and Walker, K.J. (1989). LH-RH analogues in breast and gynaecological cancers. *J. Steroid Biochem.*, **33**, 801–4

12. Walker. K.J., Turkes, A., Williams, M., Blamey, R.W. and Nicholson, R.I. (1986). Preliminary endocrinological evaluation of sustained-release formulation of the LH-releasing hormone agonist D-Ser (Bu')[6] Azgly[10] LH-RH in premenopausal women with advanced breast cancer. *J. Endocrinol.*, **111**, 349–53

13. Klijn, J.G.M. and De Jong, F.H. (1987). Long-term LH-RH agonist (Buserelin) treatment in metastatic premenopausal breast cancer. In Klijn, J.G.M., Paridens, R. and Foekens, J.A. (eds.) *Hormonal Manipulation of Cancer*, pp. 343–52. (New York: Raven Press)

14. Harvey, H.A. (1988). Luteinizing hormone-releasing hormone agonist in the therapy of breast cancer. In Osborne, C.K. (ed.) *Endocrine Therapies in Breast and Prostate Cancer*, pp. 39–50. (Boston: Kluwer Academic Publishers)

15. Vermeulen, A. (1976). The hormonal activity of the postmenopausal ovary. *J. Clin. Endocr. Metab.*, **42**, 247–53

16. Beksac, M.S., Kisnisci, H.A., Cakar, A.N. and Beksac, M. (1983). The endocrinological evaluation of bilateral and unilateral oophorectomy in premenopausal women. *Int. J. Fertil.*, **28**, 219–24

17. Nicholson, R.I., Walker, K.J., Turkes, A. *et al.* (1987). The British Experience with the LH-RH agonist Zoladex (ICI 118630) in the treatment of Breast Cancer. In Klijn, J.G.M., Paridens, R. and Foekens, J.A. (eds.)

Hormonal Manipulation of Cancer, pp. 331–41. (New York: Raven Press)

18. Harvey, H.A., Lipton, A. and Max, D.T. (1987). LH-RH agonist treatment of breast cancer; a phase II study in the USA. In Klijn, J.G.M., Paridens, R. and Foekens, J.A. (eds.) *Hormonal Manipulation of Cancer,* pp. 321–30. (New York: Raven Press)

19. Williams, M.R., Walker, K.J., Turkes, A., Elston, C.W., Blamey, R.W. and Nicholson R.I. (1986). The use of an LH-RH agonist (ICI 118630, Zoladex) in advanced premenopausal breast cancer. *Br. J. Cancer*, **53**, 629–36

20. Williams, M. and Nicholson, R.I. (1986). The premenopausal women: treatment of secondary breast cancer. In Blamey, R.W. (ed.) *Complications in the Management of Breast Disease*, pp. 128–36. (London: Bailliere Tindall)

21. Williamson, K., Robertson, J.F.R., Ellis, I.O., Elston, C.W., Nicholson, R.I. and Blamey, R.W. (1988). Effect of LH-RH agonist, Zoladex on ovarian histology. *Br. J. Surg.*, **75**, 595–6

22. Dulfour, J., Cahill, L.P. and Maulean, P. (1979). Short and long-term effects of hypophysectomy and unilateral ovariectomy on ovarian follicular populations in sheep. *J. Reprod. Fertil.*, **57**, 301–9

23. Hirshfield, A.N. (1985). Comparison of granulosa cell proliferation in small follicles of hypophysectomized, prepubertal and mature rats. *Biol. Reprod.*, **32**, 979–87

24. Kardinal, C.G. and Donegan, W.L. (1979). Endocrine and hormonal therapy. In Donegan, W.L. and Spratt, V.S. (eds.) *Cancer of the Breast* 2nd Edn., vol. 5 in the series *Major Problems in Clinical Surgery*, pp. 361–404. (London: W.B. Saunders Company)

25. Taylor, S.G. (1962). Endocrine ablation in disseminated mammary carcinoma. *Surg. Gynecol. Obstet.*, **115**, 443–8

26. Fracchia, A.A., Farrow, J.H., DePalo, A.J., Connolly, D.P. and Huvos, A.G. (1969). Castration for primary inoperable or recurrent breast carcinoma. *Surg. Gynecol. Obstet.*, **128**, 1226–34

27. Lee, Y.T. and Hori, J.M. (1971). Significance of ovarian metastasis in therapeutic oophorectomy of advanced breast cancer. *Cancer*, **27**, 1374–8

28. Walker, K.J., Turkes, A., Robertson, J.F.R., Blamey, R.W., Griffiths, K. and Nicholson, R.I. (1989). Endocrine effects of combination antioestrogen and LH-RH agonist therapy in premenopausal advanced breast cancer patients. *Eur. J. Cancer Clin. Oncol.*, **25**, 651–4

29. Klijn, J.G.M., Van Geel, A.N., Sandow, J. and De Jong, F.H. (1988). Treatment with high dose LH-RH agonist (Buserelin) plus tamoxifen and with buserelin implants in premenopausal patients; an endocrine and pharmacokinetic study. In Bresciani, F., King, R.J.B., Lippman, M.E. and Raynaud, J.-P. (eds.) *Progress in Cancer Research and Therapy* Vol. 35, *Hormones and Cancer*, 3, pp. 365–8. (New York: Raven Press)

3

Clinical experience with Zoladex in the United Kingdom

R.W. Blamey

CLINICAL STUDIES

Breast cancer

Zoladex was originally assessed as a daily subcutaneous injection and later as a depot formulation given once a month by subcutaneous injection into the abdominal wall. Our first study was performed in patients with stage III and IV breast cancer who had no previous endocrine therapy or chemotherapy. Fifty-three patients were entered of whom 45 were evaluable for response. Response was assessed by UICC criteria but in addition the response had to last for a period of at least 6 months to be acceptable. For this reason our response rates are a little lower than those generally quoted in the endocrine response literature. During the early period of the study surgical oophorectomy was performed after disease progression on Zoladex. This was performed because Zoladex was experimental and surgical oophorectomy was the standard treatment at that time. Later, when it became apparent that Zoladex gave complete ovarian suppression this procedure was omitted. The endocrinological data from this trial are outlined in Williams *et al.* [1].

Of the 45 evaluable women, 14 (31%) had a complete or partial response to Zoladex which is similar to the figure we would expect from surgical oophorectomy. Apart from two patients who developed skin rashes, the side-effects were symptoms that would be expected in menopausal women only.

Twenty-six patients had a surgical oophorectomy after response and later progression or if they progressed with no evidence of response. Twenty-four patients were assessable for response after surgery and four (15%) responded all of whom had not responded to Zoladex. Three of these, all with bone metastases, had a very early change of therapy and it is clear they did not receive treatment for long enough to evaluate response to Zoladex. The other patient was refractory to Zoladex and had recurrent oestradiol peaks during the 6-month treatment period. This patient was given daily subcutaneous injection: we have not seen this problem with the depot formulation.

We conclude that the clinical and endocrinological responses to Zoladex are similar to those seen after surgical oophorectomy[2]. Zoladex is easily administered and without specific side-effects. We now think it is the treatment of choice for premenopausal women with advanced breast cancer. It may not be licensed for use until superiority or equivalence with surgical treatments is shown in phase III trials.

Trials are now in progress to assess the therapeutic value of a combination of tamoxifen and Zoladex compared with tamoxifen alone. The theoretical disadvantage of the combined treatment is that in the reduced oestrogenic environment produced by Zoladex-induced ovarian suppression tamoxifen may act as an agonist. The combination reduces oestradiol to a significantly greater extent than Zoladex alone. Trials under way in Europe will determine whether the combination has therapeutic advantage in premenopausal patients with advanced breast cancer. Trials of Zoladex in postmenopausal patients show only low response rates and the drug does not appear to be useful in this clinical situation.

Benign breast disease

A recent study suggests that Zoladex may be of value for the treatment of benign breast disease. Twenty-one women with marked breast pain sufficient to interfere with their quality of life and who were refractory to treatment with danazol were included. The pain was cyclical in some patients. After 6 months of treatment with Zoladex symptom relief was assessed as significant in 17 of 21 (8%)[3]. However, 10 patients had required another 6-month course. The side-effects were those of the menopause but no patient asked to stop therapy. In Nottingham 10 patients with cyclical breast pain were treated, often with marked symptomatic relief. The two studies suggest that Zoladex may be a useful therapy for cyclical mastalgia resistant to standard therapies.

EFFECT OF ZOLADEX ON HISTOLOGY OF THE OVARIES

The histological appearances of the ovaries removed from 23 women who were ovariectomized after Zoladex therapy were compared with those from 34 women ovariectomized as first endocrine therapy. The number of follicles present was similar in each group but Zoladex resulted in reduced follicular maturation. More cysts were seen in the Zoladex group but the numbers of corpora lutea were similar.

CONCLUSION

Zoladex and other luteinizing hormone releasing hormone agonists are a major therapeutic advance and should supplant surgical oophorectomy for the treatment of advanced breast cancer. It is likely that they will be useful as an adjuvant therapy in premenopausal breast cancer and for benign breast disease resistant to standard therapies.

REFERENCES

1. Williams, M.R., Walker, K.J., Turkes, A., Blamey, R.W. and Nicholson, R.I. (1986). The use of an LH-RH agonist (ICI 118630, Zoladex) in advanced premenopausal breast cancer. *Br. J. Cancer*, **53**, 629–36
2. Hamed, H., Caleffi, M., Chaudary, M.A., Fentiman, I.S. (1990). An open study: LHRH analogue for treatment of recurrent and refractory mastalgia. *Ann. Surg.*, submitted
3. Walker, K.J., Walker, R.F., Turkes, A., Robertson, J.F.R., Blamey, R.W., Griffiths, K. and Nicholson, R.I. (1989). Endocrine effects of combination antioestrogen and LH-RH agonist therapy in premenopausal patients with advanced breast cancer. *Eur. J. Cancer Clin. Oncol.*, **25**, 651–4

4

GnRH analogues in pre- and perimenopausal advanced breast cancer: German clinical experience with Zoladex

*M. Kaufmann**

INTRODUCTION

Different aims in the treatment of metastatic breast cancer were stated by the members of a Consensus Development Conference in 1988[1] (Table 1). Aims in clinical trials are: to prolong time to treatment failure, to increase response rates, and to improve quality of life. The aim for physicians in practice should be the attempt to achieve maximal palliation of symptoms with minimal toxicity (time to progression). Most patients should start with endocrine treatment as their first mode of therapy in low risk situations (selection criteria: hormone receptors, disease-free interval, sites and number of metastases). Among premenopausal women oophorectomy remains the classical initial treatment[2] (Figure 1).

The development of gonadotropin releasing hormone (GnRH) analogues[3,4] now offers the possibility of a medical castration. Even the application of a long-acting depot formulation, which has been studied since 1984 offers the advantage of better patient compliance compared to daily applications[5–7].

---

* on behalf of the Cooperative Zoladex Study Group.

Table 1 Aims of therapy of metastatic breast cancer (Consensus Development Conference 7/1988 Munich[1])

A. In clinical trials:
- to prolong time to treatment failure
- to increase response rate
- to improve quality of life

B. For physicians in practice:
- to achieve maximum palliation of symptoms with minimum toxicity for a time as long as possible (time to progression)

ᴄASES OF CARCINOMA OF THE MAMMA. [JULY 11, 1896.

red.
ːade
› bc
age.
ars;
It
ʌave
is to
ase ?
ose ?
ˈlace
ɪn in
ːsion
that
ɪses,
ɪ of
ːical
any
hese
ʊres
ˌtary
ᵹ tɔ

ON THE TREATMENT OF INOPERABLE CASES OF CARCINOMA OF THE MAMMA: SUGGESTIONS FOR A NEW METHOD OF TREATMENT, WITH ILLUSTRATIVE CASES.[1]

By GEORGE THOMAS BEATSON, M.D. EDIN.,

SURGEON TO THE GLASGOW CANCER HOSPITAL; ASSISTANT SURGEON, GLASGOW WESTERN INFIRMARY; AND EXAMINER IN SURGERY TO THE UNIVERSITY OF EDINBURGH.

I HAVE no doubt it has fallen to the lot of nearly every medical man to have been consulted from time to time by patients suffering from carcinoma so widely spread or so situated that it has been quite apparent that nothing in the way of operative measures could be recommended. Such cases naturally excite our sympathy, but they also bring home to us the fact that once a case of cancer has passed

Figure 1 First report of inoperable cases of the mamma with oophorectomy in *The Lancet* 1896

The objectives of the German phase II pilot and multicentre studies, which were performed in pre- and perimenopausal low-risk patients with metastatic breast cancer were:

(1) to evaluate the endocrine effects;
(2) to determine objective response rates and duration of response; and,
(3) to register side-effects of this new treatment modality.

28

This report presents the interim results of the German Zoladex Trial, an open phase II multicentre study started in 1984, and the results of patients treated in Heidelberg with second- or third-line hormonal therapy after Zoladex first-line treatment.

MATERIAL AND METHODS

Patients

In total 134 women entered the trial of whom 118 were evaluable. The reasons for ineligibility ($n = 16$) are listed in Table 2. All patients were pre- or perimenopausal (median age 42 years, range 25–55) with histologically proven metastatic breast carcinoma and measurable disease. Distant metastatic lesions were located in bone ($n = 45$), viscera ($n = 20$), loco-regional ($n = 16$) and multiple sites ($n = 37$). Median disease-free interval was 18 months (range 0–109). Sixty-eight patients had no adjuvant or palliative pretreatment, 42 adjuvant cytotoxic and nine adjuvant tamoxifen therapy (one patient had both adjuvant therapies). Informed consent was obtained from all patients prior to therapy.

Table 2 Patient evaluability in advanced premenopausal breast cancer: German Zoladex Trial

	n
No. of patients	134
Evaluable	118
Non-evaluable	16
non-advanced	4
postmenopausal	2
other concomitant malignancy	1
additional systemic treatment	5
adjuvant chemotherapy not finished > 6 months	1
lost to follow-up	3

Therapy

Zoladex (3.6 mg), a GnRH agonist in a depot formulation, was administered subcutaneously every 28 days into the lower abdominal wall without local anaesthesia. In total 1105 applications were given.

Steroid hormone receptors

Biochemical oestrogen (ER) and progesterone (PR) receptor determinations were performed according to the EORTC-criteria[8]. Sixty-nine and 64 patients presented with an ER- or PR-positive tumour, 24 and 25 patients with an ER- or PR-negative tumour, respectively. ER or PR status was unknown in 25 and 29 patients, respectively.

Follow-up and response criteria

Clinical examination and blood chemistry were determined every 4 weeks at the time of Zoladex injections. Lung X-ray, bone scintigraphy, ultrasound of the liver and X-ray of bone lesions were performed every 3 months.

Objective response (CR, complete response; PR, partial response; NC, no change; and P, progression) was determined according to UICC criteria[9] with a minimum follow-up time of more than 3 months. Patients with a shorter time on therapy were judged as having primary progression.

RESULTS

Systemic endocrine effects

Luteinizing hormone and follicle stimulating hormone levels were significantly suppressed by Zoladex. Mean oestradiol values fell into the range of castrate level within 3 weeks of therapy and this suppression was maintained for the duration of therapy, even for more than 2 years[10].

Subjective response

Seventy-seven patients showed symptoms before Zoladex treatment. Subjective response (relief of bone pain, improvement of performance status) occurred in 53 (69%) of them.

Objective response

Overall objective tumour response and duration of response are given in Table 3. CR+PR was seen in 53 (44.9%), and NC in 33 (27.7%) of the 118 evaluable patients. Median time to response was 4 months (range 2–11). Median duration of response was 8+ months (range 2–24+).

Median duration of Zoladex therapy was 11 months (range 1–30). In Figure 2 'time to progression' (Kaplan–Meier Estimation) dependent on best response (CR, PR, NC, P) with a minimum follow-up time of more than 3 months is shown.

Table 4 shows response rates related to different sites of metastases. Loco-regional metastases responded best (10/16), followed by bone (21/45), visceral (9/20) and multiple (13/37) metastases.

An objective response was shown by 49.3% and 45.3% of the patients with ER- or PR-positive tumours, 33.3% and 48% of the patients with ER- or PR-negative tumours and 41.4% and 41.4% of patients with ER or PR unknown tumours, respectively. Figure 3 shows the 'time to progression' dependent on the steroid hormone receptor status.

Table 3 Zoladex depot in premenopausal patients with metastatic breast cancer ($n = 118$): overall objective response, duration of response and time to progression

Response	n	(%)	Duration of response (months)		Time to progression (months)	
			range	(median)	range	(median)
CR	12	(10.2)	3–24+	(10+)	6–29	(13+)
PR	41	(34.7) } (44.9)	2–19+	(5+)	5–30	(8+)
NC	33	(28.0)	2–22+	(6+)	4–22+	(6+)
P	32	(27.1)	1– 3	(2)	1– 3	(2)
Total	118	(100)				

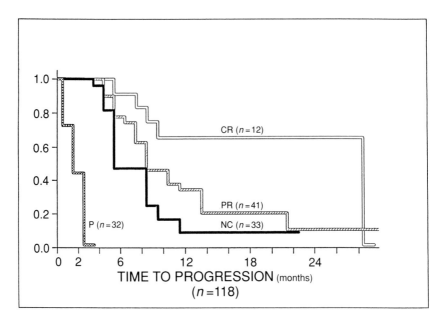

Figure 2 Zoladex depot in premenopausal patients with advanced breast cancer (*n* = 118). Kaplan–Meier estimation: 'time to progression' dependent on best response (CR, PR, NC) with a minimum follow-up of more than 3 months. All other patients were judged as P

Table 4 Zoladex depot in premenopausal patients with metastatic breast cancer (*n* = 118): response rates in relation to the metastatic tumour sites

| | *Metastatic tumour sites* | | | | |
Response	*Bone*	*Local*	*Visceral*	*Multiple*	*Total*
CR	3	5	3	1	12
PR	18	5	6	12	41
NC	15	2	5	11	33
P	9	4	6	13	32
Total	45	16	20	37	118

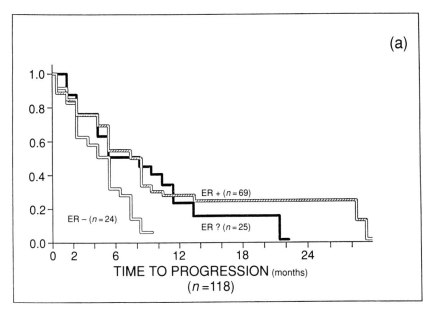

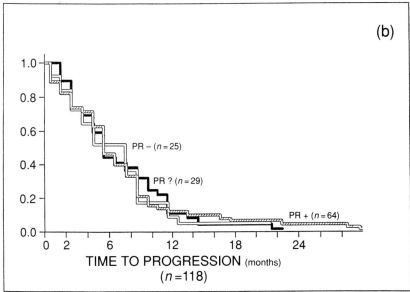

Figure 3 Zoladex depot in premenopausal patients with advanced breast cancer (*n* = 118). Kaplan–Meier estimation: 'time to progression' dependent on the steroid hormone receptor status (+, positive; –, minus; ?, unknown); (a) oestrogen receptor status, (b) progesterone receptor status

More patients with a disease-free interval (DFI) of > 2 years responded to therapy (53.1%) compared to those with a DFI of ≤ 2 years (39.1%). In Figure 4 the 'time to progression' dependent on DFI is shown. The difference between DFI > 2 and DFI ≤ 2 years is significant with a p value of 0.05 (log rank test).

Side-effects

Zoladex was well tolerated without serious toxicity. No patient was withdrawn due to an adverse reaction.

In total all 1105 applications were given without complications. Moderate itching at the place of injection site occurred in only 0.5% of all cases.

All patients were amenorrhoeic after one to two applications (4–8 weeks). Two patients had still one menstruation after 5 months, but in one case the depot application was 2 weeks too late. Three patients had spotting.

Due to the pharmacological effects of Zoladex, hot flushes were expected and they were noted in 84 patients. Two patients were depressed and two complained of nausea. Other side-effects were only seen in single cases (depression, migraine, hypotension, sleep disturbances, feeling of fullness in the breasts, oedema of eyelid, stiffness of hands). Also only one patient showed an increased bone pain for 6 weeks.

Zoladex in combination with other additive endocrine treatment

First encouraging results were achieved with second-line (tamoxifen, Nolvadex) and even third-line (aminoglutethimide) hormonal therapy after progression during Zoladex first-line therapy for patients who initially responded (Table 5). CR, PR and NC was seen in 10/15 patients, receiving additional tamoxifen (30 mg/day) to Zoladex as second-line therapy. In third-line treatment (Zoladex plus aminoglutethimide) all five women responded with one with PR (1) and four with NC (4).

These combination therapies were also well tolerated without severe toxicities. Based on more and longer experience with these hormonal combinations new sequential treatment scheme will be proposed for premenopausal women with metastatic breast cancer.

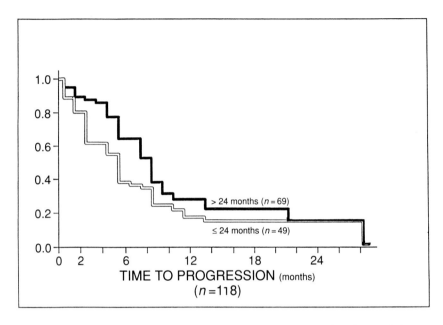

Figure 4 Zoladex depot in premenopausal patients with advanced breast cancer ($n = 118$). Kaplan–Meier estimation: 'time to progression' dependent on disease-free interval of ≤ 2 years and > 2 years ($p = 0.05$)

Table 5 Early results of response to second- and third-line hormonal therapy during continuation of Zoladex in patients treated in Heidelberg

	n	*CR*	*PR*	*NC*	*P*
Second-line hormonal therapy (Zoladex + Nolvadex)					
Response	15	0	3	7	5
Time to progression (months) range (median)			6–17 (13)	4–27 (7)	< 3
Third-line hormonal therapy (Zoladex + aminoglutethimide)					
Response	5	0	1	4	0
Time to progression (months) range (median)		—	—	2–8 (7)	—

DISCUSSION

About one third of all metastatic breast cancer patients respond to endocrine treatment (Table 6). The response is directly correlated to steroid hormone receptors. In premenopausal low-risk patients with metastatic breast cancer oophorectomy is still standard care. However, this form of treatment is combined with a high rate of morbidity (e.g. psychological trauma of a definitive castration, surgical risk). GnRH analogues now offer the possibility of an effective and reversible castration. Drug-induced castration with GnRH analogues yielded even higher response rates for collected data in the literature than oophorectomy (Table 6). However, this may be due to patient selection. Chronic administration of GnRH analogues results, after an initial stimulation of sex steroid production, in down-regulation of the GnRH receptor, inhibition of gonadotropin release and resultant suppression of ovarian hormone production, the 'medical castration'.

Objective remission rates between 31 and 60% with different GnRH analogues in various formulations are reported in the literature[5-7,11-15].

First results with the depot formulation of Zoladex have been described by Williams et al.[15], Wander et al.[16] and Kaufmann et al.[6]. This new drug with its elegant form of application produced effective castration and response rates at least as good as surgical castration. In this series overall objective response and duration is related to an ER-positive steroid hormone receptor status. However clinical response was also seen in ER-negative patients. This fact may be due to a direct effect of Zoladex on

Table 6 Endocrine response data from comprehensive reviews[19]

Treatment	n	Response rates CR+PR (%)
Ovariectomy	1674	33
Tamoxifen	3988	32
Aminoglutethimide	1153	31
Glucocorticoids	756	25
Medroxyprogesterone acetate	1175	33
Megestrol acetate	810	29
GnRH analogues	258	43

breast cancer cells in addition to the known endocrine alterations in the patient. Evidence for a direct antitumour effect are suggested by the identification of GnRH receptors in breast cancer tissue[17]. Further evidence has been suggested by an *in vitro* study showing a retardation in growth of cultured mouse mammary tumour cells after the application of a GnRH agonist[18]. Another possibility is that the receptor assay was falsely negative in these patients (determinations partly more than 9 years ago). Responses seen in ER-negative patients were also reported with other GnRH analogues[11].

The side-effects relating to Zoladex therapy were minimal and all patients tolerated treatment well.

Therapy modalities available today to treat patients with metastatic breast cancer have increased substantially. A new adequate sequence of endocrine therapy in low-risk situations of metastatic breast cancer is shown in Figure 5 according to menopausal status of the patients. In premenopausal women

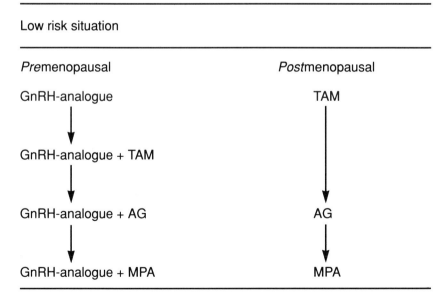

Figure 5 Sequence of endocrine therapy in metastatic breast cancer patients in a low-risk situation; TAM, tamoxifen; AG, aminoglutethimide; MPA, medroxyprogesterone acetate

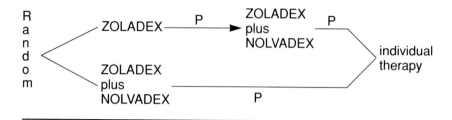

Figure 6 International study design for the treatment of metastatic breast cancer in pre- and perimenopausal patients

oophorectomy should be replaced by treatment with GnRH analogues. Further investigations will elicit if Zoladex alone or in combination with other hormonal therapies (e.g. tamoxifen) (Figure 6) is superior as a first line therapy in the management of metastatic breast cancer.

For new modalities of breast cancer treatment and new ways of delivering conventional therapy, the participants of the 1988 Consensus Development Conference[1] should urge physicians to enroll their patients in a clinical trial.

REFERENCES

1. Consensus Statement (1989). In Kaufmann, M., Henderson, I.C. and Enghofer, E. (eds.) *Therapeutic Management of Metastatic Breast Cancer Consensus Development in Cancer Therapy 1*, pp. 81–5. (Berlin, New York: De Gruyter)
2. Beatson, G.T. (1896). On the treatment of inoperable cases of carcinoma of the mamma: Suggestions for a new method of treatment with illustrative cases. *Lancet*, **ii**, 104–7
3. Furr, B. (1983). ICI 118 630 ein LH–RH–Analogon zur Behandlung des Mamma- und Prostatakarzinoms. In Kubli, F., Nagel, G.F., Kadach, U. and Kaufmann, M. (eds.) *Neue Wege in der Brustkrebsbehandlung*, pp. 243–52. (Munich: Zuckschwerdt)
4. Schally, A.V., Redding, T.W. and Cumaru-Schally, A.M. (1984). Potential use of analogs of luteinizing hormone-releasing hormones in the treatment of hormone-sensitive neoplasm. *Cancer Treat. Rep.*, **68**, 281–9

5. Höffken, K., Miller, B., Fischer, P. *et al.* (1986). Buserelin in treatment of premenopausal advanced breast cancer. Abstracts of the *International Symposium on Hormonal Manipulation of Cancer*, Rotterdam, 4–6 June 1986. *Eur. J. Cancer Clin. Oncol.*, **22**, 746

6. Kaufmann, M., Schmid, H., Kiesel, L. *et al.* (1988). GnRH-Agonisten (Zoladex)-Therapie bei prämenopausalen Frauen mit metastasierendem Mammakarzinom. *Geburtsh. u. Frauenheilk.*, **48**, 528–32

7. Klijn, J.G.M., de Jong, F.H., Lamberts, S.W.J. and Blankenstein, M.A. (1985). LHRH-agonist treatment in clinical and experimental human breast cancer. *J. Steroid Biochem.*, **23**, 867–73

8. EORTC Breast Cancer Cooperative Group (1973). Standards for the assessment of estrogen receptors in human breast cancer. *Eur. J. Cancer*, **9**, 379–81

9. Hayward, J.L., Carbone, P.O., Heuson, J.-C. *et al.* (1977). Assessment of response to therapy in advanced breast cancer. *Cancer*, **39**, 1289–94

10. Kaufmann, M., Jonat, W., Kleeberg, U. *et al* (1989). Goserelin, a depot gonadotrophin-releasing hormone agonist in the treatment of premenopausal patients with metastatic breast cancer. *J. Clin. Oncol.*, **7**, 1113–19

11. Harvey, H.A., Lipton, A., Max, D.T. *et al.* (1985). Medical castration produced by the GnRH analogue leuprolide to treat metastatic breast cancer. *J. Clin. Oncol.*, **3**, 1068–72

12. Höffken, K., Becker, R., Kurschel, E. *et al.* (1988). Buserelin in the treatment of premenopausal patients with advanced breast cancer. In Höffken, K. (ed.) *LH-RH Agonists in Oncology*, pp. 149–62. (Berlin: Springer)

13. Klijn, J.G.M. (1984). Long-term LHRH-agonist treatment in metastatic breast cancer as single treatment and in combination with other additive endocrine treatments. *J. Med. Oncol. Tumour Pharmacother.*, **1**, 123–8

14. Manni, A., Santen, R., Harvey, H. *et al.* (1986). Treatment of breast cancer with gonadotropin-releasing hormone. *Endocr. Rev.*, **7**, 89–94

15. Williams, M.R., Walker, K.J., Türkes, A. *et al.* (1986). The use of an LH-RH agonist (ICI 118630, Zoladex) in advanced premenopausal breast cancer. *Br. J. Cancer*, **53**, 629–36

16. Wander, H.E., Kleeberg, U.R., Schachner-Wünschmann, E. and Nagel, G.A. (1987). A long-acting depot preparation of a synthetic GnRH agonist (Zoladex) in the treatment of pre- and postmenopausal advanced breast cancer (BC). Abstract *3rd International Congress on Hormones and Cancer*, Hamburg, 6–11 September, 1987

17. Kiesel, L., Kaufmann, M., Haesler, F. *et al* (1988). GnRH-Rezeptoren im menschlichen Mammakarzinomgewebe. *Geburtsh. u. Frauenheilk.*, **48**, 420–24

18. Corbin, A. (1982). From contraception to cancer: A review of the therapeutic application of LH-RH analogues as antitumour agents. *Yale J. Br. Med.*, **55**, 27–47

19. Rose, C. (1989). Endocrine therapy of advanced breast cancer. In Kaufmann, M., Henderson, I.C. and Enghofer, E. (eds.) *Therapeutic Management of Metastatic Breast Cancer*, pp. 3–17. (Berlin, New York: De Gruyter)

APPENDIX

Cooperative German Zoladex Study Group

Institution	Participants
UFK Heidelberg	Kaufmann, Schmid, Kubli
UFK Hamburg	Jonat, Kunz, Maass
Hämat. Onk. Praxis Hamburg	Kleeberg
UFK Großhadern München	Eiermann, Hepp
UFK Rechts d. Isar München	Jänicke, Graeff
FK Med. Hoch. Hannover	Schwarzenau, Hilfrich
UFK Mainz	Gerlach, Kreienberg
UFK Homburg/Saar	Strunz, Bastert
UFK Frankfurt	Albrecht, Schmidt-Matthiessen
UFK Steglitz Berlin	Scheiber, Weitzel
Univ.-Klinik, Onkol, Göttingen	Wander, Nagel
Marienhospital Osnabrück	Brunnert
UFK Marburg	Schmidt-Rhode, Schulz
KH Barmh. Brüder, Onk. Regensburg	Wellens
UFK Freiburg	Kleine, Pfleiderer
Ärztegem. Paderborn	Hegemann
KH Neu-Bethesda, FK Hannover	Corterier

5

A possible direct action of a GnRH agonist, Zoladex, on *in vitro* clonogenic growth of human breast cancer

Y. Nomura, H. Tashiro and K. Hisamatsu

It has been generally accepted that the effects of gonadotropin releasing hormone (GnRH) agonists are mediated by the inhibition of gonadotropin release followed by a decrease in circulating oestrogens[1,2]. However, it has been recently reported that the GnRH agonists may have a direct action on the cell growth of breast cancer: there is evidence of significant regression of breast cancer tumours in postmenopausal patients[3-5], the cell growth inhibition of a human breast cancer cell line by this agent[6], and also the presence of specific binding affinity or specific receptors to the GnRH on the plasma membrane of cancer cells[7,8].

In this report, we describe the effects of a GnRH agonist, Zoladex, on the clonogenic growth of a human breast cancer cell line, MCF-7 on plastic dishes, and its effects on *in vitro* clonogenic growth in soft agar of human primary breast cancer cells.

MATERIALS AND METHODS

Colony formation of MCF-7 cells on plastic dishes

A hormone responsive human breast cancer cell line, MCF-7 was provided from the Mason Research Institute (Rockville, USA) and has been cultured in this laboratory. MCF-7 cells were dispersed with trypsin and 400 to 800 cells were plated on each 60 mm Nunc plastic dish. After 24 hours, various concentrations of Zoladex, 10^{-10}M to 10^{-5}M were added to the medium. The experiments were performed in parallel in the presence or absence of oestradiol-17β (E_2: 10^{-8}M) in the medium. After incubation for 2 weeks, the dishes were stained and the number of colonies was counted.

The foetal calf sera (FCS) used in this experiment were treated with dextran-coated charcoal (DCC) at 45°C, in order to decrease the endogenous steroid hormone levels, including oestrogens.

In vitro clonogenic assay in soft agar of human breast cancer

Primary breast cancers without prior treatment were biopsied or removed from the resected specimens at the time of mastectomy, and dissected from the surrounding normal or fat tissues. Tumour tissues were minced and centrifuged at 1000 rpm for 10 min. The pellets were washed twice, and mixed with an enzyme-disperse medium (RPMI 1640 with 10% DCC-treated FCS, insulin and 0.7% collagenase) for 30 min, at 37°C, being agitated by a stirrer. The cells were than filtered through a stainless steel mesh. These single cells were cultured in a bilayer agar system as described by Hamburger and Salmon[9]. Between 2×10^5 and 5×10^5 cells were pipetted onto each dish and incubated at 37°C in a 5% CO_2, 100% humidified atmosphere.

Colony counts were made on the 14th day after plating. Aggregates of 30 cells or more were considered colonies[10]. Cultures of untreated controls (DCC-treated FCS alone) were compared with E_2, 10^{-8}M, tamoxifen, 10^{-6}M, and Zoladex, 10^{-6}M, separately. Only cultures with 30 or more colonies per dish were used. Estrogen (ER) and progesterone (PR) receptors were assayed in the adjacent cancer tissues using the DCC method. Measurements of 3 fmol per mg of protein of specific binding sites or more were considered to be positive.

RESULTS

Effects of Zoladex on the clonogenic growth of MCF-7 cells on plastic dishes

Escalating doses of Zoladex, from 10^{-10}M to 10^{-5}M were added to the control medium with and without E_2 at 10^{-8}M. In the dose–response curves as shown in Figure 1, there were no significant effects of Zoladex on the cell growth of MCF-7 cells in the presence or absence of E_2. In R-27 cells, a tamoxifen-resistant subline of MCF-7 cells, we could not find any effects on the clonogenic growth under these experimental conditions (data not shown).

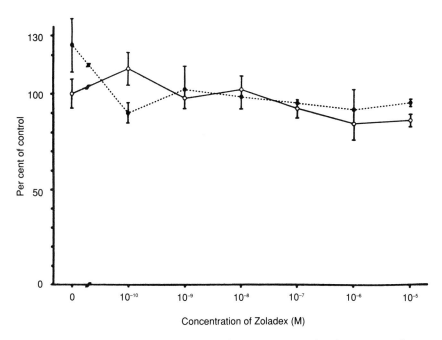

Figure 1 Effects of Zoladex on the clonogenic growth of MCF-7 cells on plastic dishes: open circles, without oestradiol; closed circles, with oestradiol; mean $\pm$ SD

Effects of Zoladex on the *in vitro* clonogenic growth in soft agar of human breast cancer

In 64 patients with primary breast cancer, there was successful colony formation (> 30 columns per dish). Details of the patients and tumours are shown in Table 1. The mean age of the patients was 53, ranging from 29 to 87. Forty-five per cent were premenopausal and 55% postmenopausal. Forty-nine (77%) of the cancers were classified to be stage I or II in the UICC system. There were 72% and 69% ER-positive and PR-positive tumours, respectively. All were identified as invasive ductal carcinoma histologically.

Table 2 indicates the responses of these primary cancers to E_2, tamoxifen and Zoladex. E_2 was shown to be effective in increasing the number of colonies per dish (mean of duplicate cultures) to 150% or more of the control in 12 of 64 cultures (19%). On the other hand, 16% or 10 of 64 cancers responded to tamoxifen or Zoladex respectively; that is, the number of colonies per dish decreased to 50% or less of the control by adding tamoxifen or Zoladex, separately in the medium.

Responses were studied in relation to the ER and PR status of the primary cancers. Eleven of 42 (26%) of ER-positive, PR-positive cancers responded to E_2, whereas only one of 16 (6%) of ER-negative, PR-negative tumours responded. This difference was not significant ($\chi^2 = 1.72$, $p = 0.19$). Similar results were obtained for tamoxifen and Zoladex in relation to inhibition of growth and receptor status (Table 2). There were no significant differences in response to these agents according to menopausal status. Responders in pre- and postmenopausal patients were shown to be 21% (6/29) and 17% (6/35) to E_2, 14% (4/29) and 17% (6/35) to tamoxifen and 10% (3/29), and 20% (7/35) to Zoladex, respectively.

The correlation between percentages of colonies to the control when treated with Zoladex and those treated with E_2 in ER-positive and ER-negative cancers is shown in Figure 2, and Figure 3 shows the correlation between Zoladex and tamoxifen. None of the correlations was significant.

Table 1 Characteristics of primary breast cancer patients

Age (yr)	52.8 ± 12.3	(29–87)
Menopausal status		
Pre–	29	(45.3%)
Post–	35	(54.7%)
Stage (UICC)		
I	5	(7.8%)
II	44	(68.7%)
IIIa	6	(9.4%)
IIIb	9	(14.1%)
ER		
+	46	(71.9%)
–	18	(28.1%)
PR		
+	44	(68.7%)
–	20	(31.2%)

Table 2 Response of primary breast cancer to oestrogen, tamoxifen or Zoladex in *in vitro* clonogenic growth in soft agar, according to ER and PR

Receptor status	E_2 ($\geq 150\%$)*		Tamoxifen ($\leq 50\%$)*		Zoladex ($\leq 50\%$)*	
ER+ PR+	26.2%	(11/42)	21.4%	(9/42)	19.0%	(8/42)
ER+ PR–	—	(0/4)	—	(0/4)	—	(0/4)
ER– PR+	—	(0/2)	—	(0/2)	—	(0/2)
ER– PR–	6.3%	(1/16)	6.3%	(1/16)	12.5%	(2/16)
Total	18.8%	(12/64)	15.6%	(10/64)	15.6%	(10/60)

*(% of control): E_2, 10^{-8}M; tamoxifen, 10^{-6}M; Zoladex, 10^{-6}M

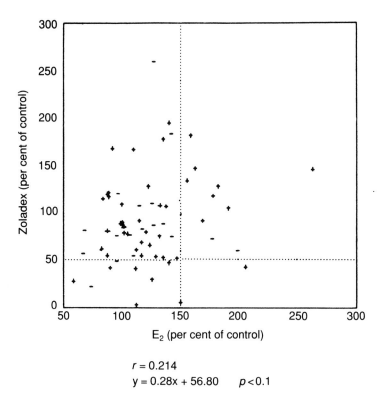

$$r = 0.214$$
$$y = 0.28x + 56.80 \qquad p < 0.1$$

Figure 2 Correlation between percentage clonogenicities of human breast cancers treated with Zoladex and those treated with E_2; +, ER–positive; –, ER–negative

DISCUSSION

Analogues of GnRH have been proved to be a significant endocrine therapy for premenopausal patients with advanced breast cancer[1,2]. The antitumour effect of the GnRH agonists is thought to be due to the suppression of the pituitary–gonadal axis[1,2]. The agents are thus indicated primarily for menstruating patients with high circulating oestrogen levels.

However, there have been some reports[3–5] in which the GnRH has induced objective regression in postmenopausal patients. Besides other possible indirect endocrine effects on postmenopausal breast cancer[4], it has been suggested that GnRH agonists may have a direct antitumour

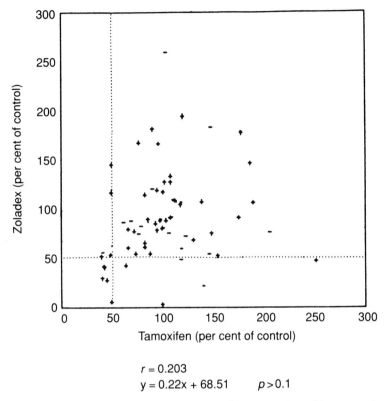

$r = 0.203$
$y = 0.22x + 68.51$ $p > 0.1$

Figure 3 Correlation between percentage clonogenicities of human primary breast cancers treated with Zoladex and those treated with tamoxifen; +, ER-positive; –, ER-negative

effect. Miller *et al.*[6] have reported that a GnRH agonist, buserelin, inhibited MCF-7 cell growth dose-dependently in culture. On the other hand, Klijn *et al.*[1] found that buserelin had a weak antioestrogenic effect on the growth of MCF-7 cells *in vitro*, without any direct effect on the cell growth. The presence of specific GnRH binding sites was reported by Eidne *et al.*[7] in all five human breast cancer cell lines tested including MCF-7 cells. However, they did not see any alteration in the cell growth *in vitro*. In the study reported here, we could not find inhibitory activity of the GnRH agonist, Zoladex on the clonogenic growth of MCF-7 cells and R-27 cells in the range of $10^{-10}M$ to $10^{-5}M$ (Figure 1). The discrepancy in these results may be due to changes in the genotype of the

MCF-7 cells, the nature of the FCS, or the method of culture.

We have used the *in vitro* clonogenic assay of primary breast cancer for the elucidation of the direct effect of a GnRH agonist, Zoladex on cell growth. The inhibitory effect of Zoladex on the clonogenicity was compared with the stimulatory effect of E_2 or inhibitory effect of tamoxifen in ER-positive and -negative cancers. There were similar percentages in responses to these three agents as shown in Table 2, although the distributions of responders and non-responders were rather different among these agents (Figures 2 and 3). These results suggest that the mechanism(s) of action of Zoladex might be different from those of E_2 or tamoxifen and that the receptors for GnRH might be differently distributed from ER and PR, making the action not via an ER system.

Although these results should be verified in more cases, the possible direct effects of the agent, even though minor, may contribute to the GnRH agonist action in pre- and postmenopausal patients with breast cancer.

REFERENCES

1. Klijn, J.G.M., De Jong, F.H., Lamberts, S.W.J. and Blankenstein, M.A. (1985). LHRH-agonist treatment in clinical and experimental human breast cancer. *J. Steroid Biochem.*, **23**, 867–73

2. Williams, M.R., Walker, K.J., Turkes, A., Blamey, R.W. and Nicholson, R.I. (1986). The use of an LH-RH agonist (ICI 118630, Zoladex) in advanced premenopausal breast cancer. *Br. J. Cancer*, **53**, 629–36

3. Plowman, P.N., Nicholson, R.I. and Walker, K.J. (1986). Remission of postmenopausal breast cancer during treatment with the luteinizing hormone releasing hormone agonist ICI 118630. *Br. J. Cancer*, **54**, 903–9

4. Schwartz, L., Guiochet, N. and Keiling, R. (1988). Two partial remissions induced by an LHRH analogue in two postmenopausal women with metastatic breast cancer. *Cancer*, **62**, 2498–500

5. Harris, A.L., Carmichael, J., Cantwell, B.M.J. and Dowsett, M. (1989). Zoladex: Endocrine and therapeutic effects in postmenopausal breast cancer. *Br. J. Cancer*, **59**, 97–99

6. Milller, W.R., Scott, W.N., Morris, R., Fraser, H.M. and Sharpe, R.M. (1985). Growth of human breast cancer cells inhibited by a luteinizing hormone-releasing hormone agonist. *Nature*, **313**, 231–3

7. Eidne, K.A., Flanagan, C.A., Harris, N.S. and Millar, R.P. (1987).

Gonadotropin-releasing hormone (GnRH)-binding sites in human breast cancer cell lines and inhibitory effects of GnRH antagonists. *J. Clin. Endocrinol. Metab.*, **64**, 425–32

8. Bützow, R., Huhtaniemi, I., Clayton, R., Wahlström, T., Andersson, L.C. and Seppälä, M. (1987). Cultured mammary carcinoma cells contain gonadotropin-releasing hormone-like immunoreactivity, GnRH binding sites and chorionic gonadotropin. *Int J. Cancer*, **39**, 498–501

9. Hamburger, A.W. and Salmon, S.E. (1977). Primary bioassay of human tumour stem cells. *Science*, **197**, 846–54

10. Nomura, Y., Tashiro, H. and Hisamatsu, K. (1989). *In vitro* clonogenic growth and metastatic potential of human operable breast cancer. *Cancer Res.*, **49**, 5288–93

6

Future trials of endocrine therapy in the management of advanced breast cancer

J.G.M. Klijn

INTRODUCTION

A lot of steroid and peptide hormones, growth factors and other trophic substances are involved in the growth regulation of breast cancer. This offers many points of action in the endocrine therapy of breast cancer both directly at the level of tumour cells or indirectly by changing the endocrine milieu. Apart from endocrine therapy there are several other systemic antitumour therapies (Table 1) of which chemotherapy is the most common. Thus far, immune therapy has not been proven to be significantly effective. But recently interferon has been shown to stimulate steroid receptor synthesis[1] and combination therapies with tamoxifen and interferons showed additive effects *in vitro*[2]. In addition, twice daily injections with γ-globulin might induce tumour growth inhibition of breast cancers found to be resistant to chemotherapy[3]. Therapies interfering with growth factor-mediated pathways and with bone (marrow)–tumour cell interaction[4-6] form a very interesting group of (potential) treatment modalities for the new future. Retinoids[7] and inhibitors of polyamine synthesis or polyamine analogues have been shown to cause tumour growth inhibition in experimental studies[8] but clinical data of studies in human breast cancer are lacking. In this paper we will present a short overview of the known systemic therapies focusing on new treatment modalities being relevant and of interest for future trials.

51

Table 1 Systemic antitumour therapies for breast cancer

1. Endocrine therapy
2. Chemotherapy
3. Immune therapy
4. Therapies interfering with growth factor-mediated pathways
5. Therapies interfering with bone (marrow)–tumour cell interaction
6. (a) Retinoids
   (b) Inhibitors of polyamine synthesis or polyamine analogues

Table 2 Endocrine therapy of breast cancer

I (1) Single treatment
      Surgical – castration
              – hypophysectomy
              – adrenalectomy

      Medical – oestrogens   : antioestrogens
              – progestins   : antiprogestins
              – androgens   : antiandrogens
              – corticosteroids   : anticorticosteroids
              – aromatase inhibitors
              – LHRH analogues
              – somatostatin analogues
              – prolactin inhibitors
  (2) Combined hormonal treatment
  (3) Alternating hormonal treatment

II (1) Combined hormonochemotherapy
  (2) Alternating hormonal (inhibitory or stimulatory)
      and chemotherapy

ENDOCRINE THERAPY

Endocrine therapy of breast cancer consists of a variety of both medical and surgical treatment modalities (Table 2). Most endocrine therapies have more than one endocrine effect frequently together with direct growth inhibitory actions. In addition, hormonal treatment can cause significant effects on autocrine and endocrine growth factor secretion and on growth factor receptor synthesis. At present, in practice, clinical interest is especially directed towards new antioestrogens, antiprogestins, new aromatase inhibitors, depot formulations of luteinizing hormone releasing hormone (LHRH) analogues, somatostatin analogues, prolactin inhibitors, endocrine combination therapies, and growth factor antagonists.

Antioestrogens

Tamoxifen is the standard first-line therapy for postmenopausal metastatic breast cancer and is even accepted as an alternative to oophorectomy in premenopausal patients. However, the stimulatory effect on the pituitary–ovarian axis in the latter group with the occurrence of sometimes very high plasma oestradiol levels is a point of concern and discussion.

At present, several new pure and steroidal antioestrogens have been developed and are under investigation in the clinic or in experimental models[9–12]. The observation that some of these new antioestrogens have growth inhibitory effects on tumour cells, being resistant for tamoxifen or even stimulated in growth by tamoxifen, is interesting[11,12]. For more extensive and detailed information on new antioestrogens refer to the chapter of Wakeling *et al.* (Chapter 12).

Antiprogestins

Antiprogestins form a new category of antihormonal agents being of potential interest in the treatment of cancer. Recently, the first antiprogestational agent, i.e. mifepristone (RU 486), which also has antiglucocorticoid properties, became available for experimental and clinical application. Initially, growth inhibitory effects on human breast cancer cells were demonstrated by extensive studies of the group of Rochefort[13] and later on by our group[14]. We also showed inhibition of tumour growth *in vivo* in rats with dimethylbenzanthracene (DMBA)-induced mammary tumours[14–18]. Recently, the first preliminary data on the effects of antiprogestin treatment of postmenopausal metastatic breast cancer were reported by Romieu et al.[19] and our group[18]. Apart from the antitumour and side-effects we investigated extensively endocrine, haematological and biochemical parameters. Mean plasma concentrations of adrenocorticotropic hormone (ACTH, $p < 0.05$), cortisol ($p < 0.001$), androstenedione ($p < 0.01$), and oestradiol ($p < 0.002$) increased significantly during treatment accompanied by a slight decrease of sex hormone binding globulin (SHBG) levels, while basal and stimulated gonadotropin levels did not change significantly. The increased basal cortisol levels could not be further stimulated by synacthen, nor suppressed by 1 mg of dexamethasone. The rise of plasma oestradiol concentrations in post-menopausal women is probably not a result of stimulation of pituitary–ovarian function (as observed in cycling female rats), but rather of stimulation of the pituitary–adrenal axis leading to an increase of the secretion of adrenal androgens, which can be used as a substrate for peripheral aromatase activity. The increase of plasma androstenedione, the positive correlation between plasma oestradiol and both cortisol ($p < 0.01$) and androstenedione ($p < 0.05$) levels, and the observation that the peak value of oestradiol in plasma was reached later than that of cortisol support this hypothesis. We observed one objective response, six instances of short-term stable disease, and four instances of progressive disease. Taking the results of our study[18] and that of Romieu et al.[19] together it appeared that mifepristone used as a second- or third-line agent caused objective remissions in four (12%) out of 33 patients and minimal response or stable disease in 15 (46%) other patients. The drug acted especially in patients with progesterone receptor (PR)-positive tumours. Interestingly, mifepristone induced remissions in advanced breast cancers that were resistant to other first-line endocrine therapies. Of potential great interest for future clinical trials is our finding that combined antioestrogenic and antiprogestational treatment blocking both oestrogen receptors (ER) and PR resulted in additive growth inhibitory effect in rat mammary tumours[17,18]. A disadvantage might be the frequent occurrence of side-effects caused by the antiglucocorticoid properties of mifepristone. Recently other antiprogestins appeared to cause tumour growth inhibition in two experimental mammary tumour models[20]. Presently, we have under investigation some new antiprogestins with less antiglucocorticoid effect and greater antitumour efficacy.

New aromatase inhibitors

The aromatase inhibitor aminoglutethimide is an effective agent in the treatment of breast cancer, but side-effects occur frequently[21,22]. Several pharmaceutical companies have developed or are developing new aromatase inhibitors. Clinical trials using 4-hydroxyandrostenedione[23] for treatment of women with breast cancer are ongoing in several centres. More recently the clinical results of a new potent non-steroidal aromatase inhibitor (CGS 16949A) without intrinsic androgenic or oestrogenic properties were published[24,25]. Using dosages ranging from 0.6 to 1.6 mg daily Santen *et al.*[24] found a degree of oestrogen reduction (35–70%) similar to that caused with much higher dosages (100-fold) of aminoglutethimide, but in the absence of side-effects. From an endocrine point of view the optimal dose appeared to be 2 mg per day. Urinary cortisol excretion did not decrease during the study but a significant blunting of plasma cortisol responses to ACTH occurred with the 16 mg daily dose. Dowsett and Lab[25] reported a decrease in plasma aldosterone levels during treatment with 2 mg CGS 16949A. In addition, Lamberts *et al.*[26] demonstrated a potent inhibition of 11ß-hydroxylase activity and of aldosterone release by adrenal cells *in vitro*. Therefore it is so far unclear whether this drug affects stress-induced cortisol release in man. Many more (comparative) studies are needed to evaluate the clinical value of this agent. For the future it is interesting to learn that already still newer imidazole derivatives are in an advanced phase of development.

Depot formulations of LHRH analogues

After our initial studies with intranasal spray[27,28] of the LHRH agonist buserelin we found that subcutaneous therapy with buserelin was more effective[29,30]. Treatment with buserelin implants (6.6 mg) once per 1–2 months appeared endocrinologically as effective as high dose (2 x 1 mg) daily injections[31]. Single LHRH agonist therapy concerning 260 premenopausal patients in eight studies caused an objective response in 42% of the patients (Table 3). The objective response rate in 139 patients with ER-positive tumours was 50%. So far the longest duration of reported response is 5 years. In postmenopausal patients the response rate is approximately 10%. These responses in postmenopausal women might

Table 3 Results of single LHRH agonist treatment of premenopausal metastastic breast cancer

Reference*	LHRH agonist	n	CR+PR
Klijn *et al.*	Buserelin	23	9 (39%)
Nicholson *et al.*	Zoladex	45	14 (31%)
Harvey *et al.*	Leuprolide	25	11 (44%)
Mathé *et al.*	D-Trp-6 LHRH	8	3 (38%)
Höffken *et al.*	Buserelin	19	8 (42%)
Wander *et al.*	Zoladex	10	6 (60%)
Kaufmann *et al.*	Zoladex	12	5 (42%)
Kaufmann *et al.*	Zoladex	118	53 (45%)
Total		260	109 (42%)

Overall objective response rate of ER-positive tumours: 70/139 (50%)
Longest duration of response: 5 years

* References taken from references 30 and 33

be explained by direct antitumour effects[32,33] of LHRH analogues and/or further decrease of plasma oestradiol levels compared with normal postmenopausal controls[31,34]. We investigated the relation between pharmacokinetics and endocrine effects of buserelin implants in six patients with severe benign mastalgia. On the first treatment day there was an initial rise in plasma and urinary buserelin levels followed by a rapid fall during the next 2 days. After a plateau phase urinary buserelin/creatinine ratios decreased slowly to a mean value of 25 μg/g creatinine 4 weeks after implantation. After the last implant injection urinary buserelin/creatinine ratios remained relatively high during more than 8 weeks followed by an exponential decrease to undetectable buserelin levels at 16–22 weeks after the last implantation. A rise of suppressed plasma oestradiol concentrations to above castrate levels was found 15–20 weeks after the last buserelin implantation at a time when urinary buserelin excretion had decreased below 0.2 μg/g creatinine.

Of great interest is the combination treatment with an LHRH agonist (suppression of ovarian oestradiol secretion) and an antioestrogen (blockade of the remaining postmenopausal plasma oestradiol concentration) aiming for 'complete oestrogen blockade'[31]. Single treatment with tamoxifen stimulates pituitary–ovarian function in premenopausal women but combined treatment with LHRH agonist implants suppressed this stimulatory effect[31,35]. Pharmacokinetic studies showed that plasma concentrations of (more than) 0.20 ng/ml resulting in urinary excretion of (more than) 5 µg/g creatinine after implantation of buserelin implants once per 8 weeks caused continuous suppression of pituitary–ovarian function in spite of the presence of tamoxifen. On the other hand, addition of tamoxifen to LHRH agonist treatment can abolish the LHRH agonist-induced tumour growth inhibition *in vitro*[32,33] or can cause adverse effects in mice with ER-negative tumours[36]. However, our preliminary data show a potential better antitumour effect in patients with metastatic breast cancer than single buserelin treatment[30]. Therefore, at present we are investigating in a randomized three-arm study (EORTC 10881) the growth inhibitory effects of buserelin implants, of tamoxifen and of the combination of both drugs. Treatment with an LHRH agonist in combination with antiprogestins[17], aromatase inhibitors or somatostatin analogues might also be of interest. For the future, trials with LHRH antagonist resulting in immediate suppression of ovarian function within 1 day can be expected.

Treatment with somatostatin analogues and prolactin inhibitors

In patients with breast cancer increased plasma levels of prolactin (PRL) and growth hormone (GH) have been demonstrated[37]. Receptors for these lactotrophic hormones have been detected in 8–72% of breast cancers[38]. Hyperprolactinaemia and increased GH levels appear unfavourable prognostic factors in patients with early or metastatic breast cancer[39–42]. GH regulates the synthesis and secretion of somatomedin-C, i.e. insulin-like growth factor 1 (IGF-1), in the liver and probably locally in multiple tissues. Besides oestradiol IGF-1 is the most potent stimulatory agent of human breast cancer cells *in vitro* and appears to be one of the most important autocrine growth factors[43]. Recently, we demonstrated significant levels of IGF-1 receptors in more than 90% of primary human breast cancers[44,45].

Single treatment with dopamine agonists (PRL inhibitors) appeared to be unsuccessful in the treatment of metastatic breast cancer[46]. In experimental models an additive tumour growth inhibitory effect of bromocriptine and progestins (medroxyprogesterone acetate, MPA) has been demonstrated[47] and a direct effect on the morphology of human breast cancer cells has been found[48]. In one clinical study the addition of bromocriptine to MPA showed a slight additive growth inhibitory effect[49], but in combination with tamoxifen another study did not show any extra beneficial effect[50]. The possible beneficial effects of suppression of PRL secretion could be overruled by growth stimulatory effects induced by GH binding to the lactogenic receptors. Therefore and also in view of growth factor secretion, simultaneous inhibition of GH and PRL might be important. Somatostatin analogues decrease GH secretion and consequently IGF-1 secretion. Receptors for somatostatin have been demonstrated in 15–36% of human primary tumours[45,51–53] and in breast cancer cell lines[54,55] suggesting the possibility of direct growth inhibitory effects. Indeed, previously we demonstrated direct growth inhibitory effects of somatostatin analogues on human breast cancer cells *in vitro*[54]. Schally *et al.* demonstrated inhibition of MT/W9A mammary tumours by somatostatin analogues in rats[55,56], but we did not observe such effects in DMBA-induced rat mammary tumours, which appear to lack somatostatin receptors. In a first preliminary clinical study Manni *et al.* showed improvement in one out of 10 heavily pretreated patients when treated with a somatostatin analogue and bromocriptine[57].

Table 4 Possible strategies for intervention in growth factor-mediated pathways

1. Identification of populations with different prognoses based on growth factor (receptor) status of tumours
2. Withdrawal of growth stimulatory growth factors
3. Administration of growth inhibitory growth factors
4. Growth factor analogues
5. Growth factor antagonists – suramin
                              – alkyl lysophospholipid derivatives
6. (a) Cytostatic drugs linked to growth factors
   (b) Radiolabeled growth factors
7. Antibodies against growth factor receptors
8. Growth factor receptor tyrosine kinase inhibitors
9. Gene therapy

Therapies interfering with growth factor-mediated pathways

The several ways of application of such an approach are summarized in Table 4. Patients with different prognoses based on growth factor (receptor) status can be selected for different forms of therapy. Plasma growth factor concentrations can be decreased by somatostatin analogues[55] or tamoxifen[58]. Potentially, the administration of the growth inhibitory growth factor transforming growth factor β (TGF-β) might inhibit breast cancer growth[43] in patients when a sufficient amount of this agent is available. Growth factor antagonists can inhibit tumour growth *in vitro* and *in vivo* by blocking growth factor receptors for their respective growth factors. In our experience suramin caused a clear dose-dependent growth inhibitory effect on human breast cancer cells *in vitro*[59]. For the future, clinical trials have to demonstrate the possible value in patients with metastatic breast cancer. Furthermore, the development of a more specific growth factor antagonist can be expected.

REFERENCES

1. Van den Berg, H.W., Leahey, W. and Lynch, M. (1986). Interferon α increases oestrogen receptor expression in the ZR-75-1 human breast cancer cell line. *Eur. J. Cancer Clin. Oncol.*, **22**, 730
2. Goldstein, D., Bushmeyer, S.M., Witt, P.L., Jordan, V.C. and Borden, E.C. (1989). Effects of type I and II interferons on cultured human breast cells: interaction with estrogen receptors and with tamoxifen. *Cancer Res.*, **49**, 2698–702
3. Staniszewski, A., Kibler, J. and Kolodziej, J. (1989). Immunotherapy with human gammaglobulin for advanced breast cancer: a preliminary report. *Book of Abstracts 5th European Conference on Clinical Oncology,* abstract, P-0958
4. Van Holten-Verzantvoort, A.T., Bijvoet, O.L.M., Cleton, F.J., Hermans, J., Kroon, H.M. and Harinck, H.I.J. (1987). Reduced morbidity from skeletal metastases in breast cancer patients during long-term biphosphonate (APD) treatment. *Lancet*, **ii**, 983–5
5. Coleman, R.E., Woll, P.J., Miles, M., Scrivener, W. and Rubens, R.D. (1988). Treatment of bone metastases from breast cancer with (3-amino-1-hydroxypropylidene)-1, 1-biphosphonate (APD). *Br. J. Cancer*, **58**, 621–5
6. Morton, A.R., Cantrill, J.A., Pillai, G.V., McMahon, A., Anderson, D.C. and Howell, A. (1988). Sclerosis of lytic bone metastases after disodium

aminohydroxypropylidene biphosphonate (APD) in patients with breast carcinoma. *Br. Med. J.*, **297**, 772–3

7. Grandilhon, P., Mélançon, R., Djiane, J. and Kelly, P.A. (1982). Comparison of ovariectomy and retinyl acetate on the growth of established 7,12-dimethyl-benz[a]anthracene-induced mammary tumors in the rat. *J. Natl. Cancer Inst.*, **69**, 447–51

8. Glikman, P., Manni, A., Demers, L. and Bartholomew, M. (1989). Polyamine involvement in the growth of hormone-responsive and -resistant human breast cancer cells in culture. *Cancer Res.*, **49**, 1371–6

9. Musgrove, E.A., Wakeling, A.E. and Sutherland, R.L. (1989). Points of action of estrogen antagonists and a clamodulin antagonist within the MCF-7 human breast cancer cell cycle. *Cancer Res.*, **49**, 2398–404

10. Robinson, S.P. and Jordan, V.C. (1989). Antiestrogenic action of toremifene on hormone-dependent, -independent, and heterogeneous breast tumor growth in the athymic mouse. *Cancer Res.*, **49**, 1758–62

11. Gottardis, M.M., Jiang, S.-Y., Jeng, M.-H. and Jordan, V.C. (1989). Inhibition of tamoxifen-stimulated growth of an MCF-7 tumor variant in athymic mice by novel steroidal antiestrogens. *Cancer Res.*, **49**, 4090–3

12. Pyrhönen, S., Valavaara, R. and Hajba, A. (1989). High dose toremifene in advanced breast cancer resistant to or relapsed with tamoxifen treatment. *Book of Abstracts 5th European Conference on Clinical Oncology*, abstract. P-0966

13. Gill, P.G., Vignon, F., Bardon, S., Derocq, D. and Rochefort, H. (1987). Difference between R 5020 and the antiprogestin RU 486 in antiproliferative effects on human breast cancer cells. *Breast Cancer Res. Treat.*, **10**, 37–45

14. Bakker, G.H., Setyono-Han, B., Henkelman, M.S., de Jong, F.H., Lamberts, S.W.J., van der Schoot, P. and Klijn, J.G.M. (1987). Comparison of the actions of the antiprogestin mifepristone (RU 486), the progestin megestrol acetate, the LHRH analog buserelin, and ovariectomy in treatment of rat mammary tumors. *Cancer Treat. Rep.*, **71**, 1021–7

15. Bakker, G.H., Setyono-Han, B., de Jong, F.H. and Klijn, J.G.M. (1987). Mifepristone in treatment of experimental breast cancer in rats. In Klijn, J.G.M., Paridaens, R. and Foekens, J.A. (eds.) *Hormonal Manipulation of Cancer: Peptides, Growth Factors, and New (Anti)steroidal Agents*, EORTC Monograph series, vol. 18, pp. 39–46. (New York: Raven Press)

16. Van der Schoot, P., Bakker, G.H. and Klijn, J.G.M. (1987). Effects of the progesterone antagonist RU486 on ovarian activity in the rat. *Endocrinology*, **121**, 1375–82

17. Bakker, G.H., Setyono-Han, B., Portengen, H., de Jong, F.H., Foekens, J.A. and Klijn, J.G.M. (1989). Endocrine and antitumor effects of combined treatment with an antiprogestin and antiestrogen or luteinizing

hormone-releasing hormone agonist in female rats bearing mammary tumors. *Endocrinology*, **125**, 1593–8

18. Klijn, J.G.M., de Jong, F.H., Bakker, G.H., Lamberts, S.W.J., Rodenburg, C.J. and Alexieva-Figusch, J. (1989). Antiprogestins, a new form of endocrine therapy for human breast cancer. *Cancer Res.*, **49**, 2851–6

19. Romieu, G., Maudelonde, T., Uhlmann, A., Pujol, H., Grenier, J., Cavalie, G., Khalaf, S. and Rochefort, H. (1987). The antiprogestin RU 486 in advanced breast cancer: preliminary clinical trial. *Bull. Cancer*, **74**, 455–61

20. Schneider, M.R., Michna, H., Nishino, Y. and El Etreby, M.F. (1989). Antitumor activity of the progesterone antagonists ZK 98.299 and RU 38.486 in the hormone-dependent MXT mammary tumor model of the mouse and the DMBA- and the MNU-induced mammary tumor models of the rat. *Eur. J. Cancer Clin. Oncol.*, **25**, 691–701

21. Alexieva-Figusch, J., de Jong, F.H., Lamberts, S.W.J., van Gilse, H.A. and Klijn, J.G.M. (1987). Endocrine effects of aminoglutethimide plus hydrocortisone versus effects of high dose of hydrocortisone alone in postmenopausal metastatic breast cancer. *Eur. J. Cancer Clin. Oncol.*, **23**, 1349–56

22. Harris, A.L., Cantwell, B.M.J., Carmichael, J., Dawes, P., Robinson, A., Farndon, J. and Wilson, R. (1989). Phase II study of low dose aminoglutethimide 250 mg/day plus hydrocortisone in advanced postmenopausal breast cancer. *Eur. J. Cancer Clin. Oncol.*, **25**, 1105–11

23. Dowsett, M., Cunningham, D.C., Stein, R.C., Evans, S., Dehennin, L., Hedley, A. and Coombes, R.C. (1989). Dose-related endocrine effects and pharmacokinetics of oral and intramuscular 4-hydroxyandrostenedione in postmenopausal breast cancer patients. *Cancer Res.*, **49**, 1306–12

24. Santen, R.J., Demers, L.M., Adlercreutz, H., Harvey, H., Santner, S., Sanders, S. and Lipton, A. (1989). Inhibition of aromatase with CGS 16949 A in postmenopausal women. *J. Clin. Endocrinol. Metab.*, **68**, 99–106

25. Dowsett, M. and Lab, A. (1988). Dose-related endocrine study of aromatase inhibitor CGS 16949 A. *J. Endocrinol.*, **119**, 123 (abstract)

26. Lamberts, S.W.J., Bruining, H.A., Marzouk, H., Zuiderwijk, J., Uitterlinden, P., Blijd, J.J., Hackeng, W.H.L. and de Jong, F.H. (1989). The new aromatase inhibitor CGS-16949A suppresses aldosterone and cortisol production by human adrenal cells *in vitro*. *J. Clin. Endocrinol. Metab.*, **69**, 896–901

27. Klijn, J.G.M. and de Jong, F.H. (1982). Treatment with a luteinizing hormone-releasing-hormone analogue (buserelin) in premenopausal patients with metastatic breast cancer. *Lancet*, **i**, 1213–16

28. Klijn, J.G.M., de Jong, F.H., Blankenstein, M.A., Docter, R., Alexieva-

Figusch, J., Blonk-van der Wijst, J. and Lamberts, S.W.J. (1984). Anti-tumor and endocrine effects of chronic LHRH agonist (buserelin) treatment with or without tamoxifen in premenopausal metastastic breast cancer. *Breast Cancer Res. Treat.*, **4**, 209–20

29. Klijn, J.G.M., de Jong, F.H., Lamberts, S.W.J. and Blankenstein, M.A. (1985). LHRH-agonist treatment in clinical and experimental human breast cancer. *J. Steroid Biochem.*, **23**, 867–73

30. Klijn, J.G.M. and Foekens, J.A. (1988). Long-term peptide hormone treatment with LHRH-agonist in metastatic breast cancer. In Santen, R. and Juhos, E. (eds.) *Endocrine-dependent Breast Cancer, Critical Assessment of Recent Advances*, pp. 92–102. (Bern: Hans Huber Publishers)

31. Klijn, J.G.M., van Geel, A.N., Sandow, J. and de Jong, F.H. (1988). Treatment with high dose LHRH-agonist (buserelin) plus tamoxifen and with buserelin implants in premenopausal patients: an endocrine and pharmacokinetic study. In Bresciani, F., King, R.J.B., Lippman, M.E. and Raynaud, J.P. (eds.) *Progress in Cancer Research and Therapy*, vol. 35, pp. 365–8. (New York: Raven Press)

32. Foekens, J.A., Henkelman, M.S., Fukkink, J.F., Blankenstein, M.A. and Klijn, J.G.M. (1986). Combined effects of buserelin, estradiol and tamoxifen on the growth of MCF-7 human breast cancer cells *in vitro*. *Biochem. Biophys. Res. Commun.*, **14**, 550–6

33. Klijn, J.G.M. and Foekens, J.A. (1989). Extrapituitary actions of GnRH analogues. In Vickery, B.H. and Lunenfeld, B. (eds.) *GnRH Analogues in Cancer and Human Reproduction, Basic Aspects*, vol. 1, pp. 71–84. (Lancaster: Kluwer Academic Publishers)

34. Dowsett, M., Cantwell, B., Anshumala, L., Jeffcoate, S.L. and Harris, A.L. (1988). Suppression of postmenopausal ovarian steroidogenesis with the luteinizing hormone-releasing hormone agonist goserelin. *J. Clin. Endocrinol. Metab.*, **66**, 672–7

35. Walker, K.J., Walker, R.F., Turkes, A., Robertson, J.F.R., Blamey, R.W., Griffiths, K. and Nicholson, R.I. (1989). Endocrine effects of combination antioestrogen and LH-RH agonist therapy in premenopausal patients with advanced breast cancer. *Eur. J. Cancer Clin. Oncol.*, **25**, 651–4

36. Szende, B., Schally, A.V., Srkalovic, G. and Comaru-Schally, A.M. (1989). Adverse effect of tamoxifen with LHRH agonist on oestrogen-receptor-negative mammary carcinoma. *Lancet*, **ii**, 222–3

37. Emerman, J.T., Leaky, M., Gout, P.W. and Bruchovsky, N. (1985). Elevated growth hormone levels in sera from breast cancer patients. *Horm. Metab. Res.*, **17**, 421–4

38. Bonneterre, J. and Peyrat, J.P. (1989). Prolactin receptors and breast cancer. *Eur. J. Cancer Clin. Oncol.*, **25**, 1121–2

39. Holtkamp, W., Nagel, G.E., Wander, H.-E., Rauschecker, H.F. and von Heyden, D. (1984). Hyperprolactinemia is an indicator of progressive disease and poor prognosis in advanced breast cancer. *Int. J. Cancer*, **34**, 323–8

40. Alexieva-Figusch, J., Blankenstein, M.A., Hop, W.C.J., Klijn, J.G.M., Lamberts, S.W.J., de Jong, F.H., Docter, R., Adlercreutz, H. and van Gilse, H.A. (1984). Treatment of metastatic breast cancer patients with different dosages of megestrol acetate; dose relations, metabolic and endocrine effects. *Eur. J. Cancer Clin. Oncol.*, **20**, 33–40

41. Alexieva-Figusch, J., de Jong, F.H., Lamberts, S.W.J., Planting, A.S.Th., van Gilse, H.A., Blankenstein, M.A., Blonk-van der Wijst, J. and Klijn, J.G.M. (1987). Alternating and combined treatment with tamoxifen and progestins in postmenopausal breast cancer. In Klijn, J.G.M., Paridaens, R. and Foekens, J.A. (eds.) *Hormonal Manipulation of Cancer: Peptides, Growth Factors and New Anti(steroidal) Agents. EORTC Monograph Series*, vol. 18, pp. 145–55. (New York: Raven Press)

42. Fentiman, I.S., Brame, K., Chaudary, M.A., Champlejohn, R.S., Wang, D.Y. and Millis, R.R. (1988). Perioperative bromocriptine adjuvant treatment for operable breast cancer. *Lancet*, **i**, 609–10

43. Lippman, M.E. (1985). Growth regulation of human breast cancer. *Clin. Res.*, **83**, 375–82

44. Foekens, J.A., Portengen, H., Janssen, M. and Klijn, J.G.M. (1989). Insulin-like growth factor-1 receptors and insulin-like growth factor-1-like activity in human primary breast cancer. *Cancer*, **63**, 2139–47

45. Foekens, J.A., Portengen, H., van Putten, W.L.J., Trapman, A.M.A.C., Reubi, J.C., Alexieva-Figusch, J. and Klijn, J.G.M. (1989). The prognostic value of receptors for insulin-like growth factor-1, somatostatin, and epidermal growth factor in human breast cancer. *Cancer Res.*, **49**, 7002–9

46. Nicholson, R.I., Walker, K.J. and Davies, P. (1986). Hormone agonists and antagonists in the treatment of hormone sensitive breast and prostate cancer. *Cancer Surv.*, **5**, 463–86

47. Dauvois, S., Spinola, P.G. and Labrie, F. (1989). Additive inhibitory effects of bromocriptine (CB-154) on dimethylbenz(a) anthracene (DMBA)-induced mammary tumors in the rat. *Eur. J. Cancer Clin. Oncol.*, **25**, 891–7

48. Polyzonis, M., Kortsaris, A. and Stravoravdi, P. (1989). The influence of bromocriptine on the ultrastructure of cultured T47D (human breast cancer) cells. *J. Submicrosc. Cytol. Pathol.*, **21**, 59–62

49. Dogliotti, L., Robustelli della Cuna, G., Di Carlo, F. and BROMPA Italian Coop. Group. (1987). Medroxyprogesterone acetate high-dose (MPA-MD) versus MPA-HD plus bromocriptine in advanced breast cancer: preliminary results of a multicentre randomized clinical trial. In

Klijn, J.G.M., Paridaens, R. and Foekens, J.A. (eds.) *Hormonal Manipulation of Cancer: Peptides, Growth Factors and New Anti(steroidal) Agents. EORTC Monograph Series*, vol. 18, pp. 183–93. (New York: Raven Press)

50. Bonneterre, J., Mauriac, L., Weber, B., Roche, H., Fargeot, P., Tubiana-Hulin, M., Sevin, M., Chollet, P. and Cappelaere, P. (1988). Tamoxifen plus bromocriptine versus tamoxifen plus placebo in advanced breast cancer: results of a double-blind multicentre clinical trial. *Eur. J. Cancer Clin. Oncol.*, **24**, 1851–3

51. Reubi, J.C., Maurer, R., von Werder, K., Torhorst, J., Klijn, J.G.M. and Lamberts, S.W.J. (1987). Somatostatin receptors in human endocrine tumors. *Cancer Res.*, **47**, 551–8

52. Papotti, M., Macri, L., Bussolati, G. and Reubi, J.C. (1989). Correlative study on neuro-endocrine differentiation and presence of somatostatin receptors in breast carcinomas. *Int. J. Cancer*, **43**, 365–9

53. Fekete, M., Wittliff, J.L. and Schally, A.V. (1989). Characteristics and distribution of receptors of [D-TRP⁶]-luteinizing hormone-releasing hormone, somatostatin, epidermal growth factor, and sex steroids in 500 biopsy samples of human breast cancer. *J. Clin. Lab. Analysis*, **3**, 137–47

54. Setyono-Han, B., Henkelman, M.S., Foekens, J.A. and Klijn, J.G.M. (1987). Direct inhibitory effects of somatostatin (analogues) on the growth of human breast cancer cells. *Cancer Res.*, **47**, 1566–70

55. Schally, A.V. (1988). Oncological applications of somatostatin analogues. *Cancer Res.*, **48**, 6977–85

56. Szende, B., Lapis, K., Redding, T.W., Srkalovic, G. and Schally, A.V. (1989). Growth inhibition of MXT mammary carcinoma by enhancing programmed cell death (apoptosis) with analogs of LH-RH and somatostatin. *Breast Cancer Res. Treat.*, **14**, 307–14

57. Manni, A., Boucher, A.E., Demers, L.M., Harvey, H.A., Lipton, A., Simmonds, M.A. and Bartholomew, A. (1989). Endocrine effects of combined somatostatin analog and bromocriptine therapy in women with advanced breast cancer. *Breast Cancer Res. Treat.*, **14**, 289–98

58. Coletti, R.B., Roberts, J.D., Devlin, J.T. and Copeland, K.C. (1989). Effects of tamoxifen on plasma insulin-like growth factor I in patients with breast cancer. *Cancer Res.*, **49**, 1882–4

59. Foekens, J.A., Stuurman-Smeets, E.M.J., Groenenboom-de Munter, I., Berns, P.M.J.J., Dorssers, L.C.J. and Klijn, J.G.M. (1989). Effects of suramin on proliferation of human breast cancer cells *in vitro. Abstract Book Third IST International Symposium on Biology and Therapy of Breast Cancer*, abstract 54

Discussion I

Professor Blamey

The *in vitro* data we have just seen are raising the possibility of a direct action of Zoladex on the tumour. Would Dr Nicholson comment.

Dr Nicholson

It is difficult to put that information up against the *in vivo* observations that apparently so few responses are seen in patients with estrogen receptor-negative tumours. Depending on how one wants to manipulate cells in culture, it is very much our experience that results can be obtained in either direction.

Professor Blamey

Something against the finding being valid was that there was no correlation between the response *in vitro* between tamoxifen and Zoladex.

Professor Nomura

We have many problems with the *in vitro* assay system because we do not know the appropriate concentration of Zoladex. But there is a possibility of direct action, and there is a specific binding site of Zoladex in some tumour systems. Also there is a report of a response in postmenopausal patients. The possibility of direct action is very minor, but it may be present.

Professor Jonat

Could Dr Nicholson comment on the gonadotropin releasing hormone (GnRH) receptors in the tumours and could he also say something about the hormone profiles in postmenopausal patients?

Dr Nicholson

Dr Klijn has much more information on GnRH binding sites in breast tumours. As I understood it, the binding sites were of a lower order of magnitude in terms of their affinity than we would expect to see in the pituitary gland, and the kind of concentrations that were often used in culture systems for GnRH were much higher than we would see in circulating levels in patients. We have not really become involved in direct actions because of those particular points, although I do know that Dr Klijn has shown some very positive results.

The original data from Miller indicated that GnRH agonists could inhibit the proliferation of MCF-7 cells and that the effects were reversed by antagonists, which gives some indication of a degree of specificity.

Dr Klijn

At least four groups have demonstrated direct positive effects *in vitro*, but it is striking that there is no homology between the results. All the groups have found clear growth inhibiting effects.

Professor Blamey

The surgical sceptic will say that there are far more things that have shown growth inhibiting effects in tumours than things that have not. Pretty well everything *in vitro* seems to retard the growth of tumours.

Dr Klijn

That may well be. I have a question related to this point. There was a clear difference in the response rate of about 20% between the UK and the German series on the same drug regimen. Could that be caused by different response criteria or by the difference in the number of patients with ER-negative tumours? I ask because a letter was recently submitted to the Lancet indicating that the combination of tamoxifen and LHRH agonist can stimulate the growth of ER-negative mouse mammary tumours, so it may be that the difference in the two sets of results can be explained by the difference in the number of ER-negative patients in the two series.

Professor Blamey

Our response rate is lower than the generally quoted responses in Nottingham because we already apply a cut-off level of 6 months response, and 30% is right on what we normally expect for response to oophorectomy in our centre.

Dr Kaufmann

I fully agree.

J.E. Varhaug

Is there any risk of a rebound effect after stopping LHRH agonist leading to supraphysiological hormone levels. Also a question with reference to benign breast disease. How many of these patients experience premature menopause after stopping Zoladex?

Dr Nicholson

With regard to the rebound effect, most of the patients who currently are on Zoladex therapy then continue on Zoladex plus another antihormonal therapy as a second-line therapy.

I do not think that particular question has been addressed in breast cancer patients but it would have been addressed in mastalgia studies. Certainly the data from the work we have been involved in with Dr Mansel have not indicated any major rebound effects.

Professor Blamey

I cannot answer for the Guy's data. In our own centre all the women have recovered their periods. Their average age is only about 40 and they are only on the drug for 6 months. It is inevitable if we start to treat women later on in their forties, and we do this for a longer period, that some will go through the natural menopause. The question whether some young women will be rendered anovular is open.

Question

Professor Blamey reports that he has asked his patients who are satisfied with 4-weekly administration. Does that mean that attempts to formulate a 3-month depot have been given up, or are people still working on it?

Professor Blamey

We are not. It is ICI who were asking our impression as to whether a 3-month depot would be more acceptable. Our patients say that it would not given that it would be a bigger implant.

Mr. B. Ball

We are still working on a 3-month depot formulation for application generally in cancer and benign conditions.

Question

Are there any data associating Zoladex with tamoxifen in experimental models of the disease that shows a synergistic effect when the two drugs are associated?

Dr Nicholson

In carcinogen-induced mammary tumours, tamoxifen produces a much lower rate of tumour remission than does Zoladex. When we add the combination the rate of tumour remission is lower. So in that particular model there is no synergistic effect to the advantage of the combination.

Section II

Management of premenopausal early stage breast cancer

7

Effects of adjuvant tamoxifen and of cytotoxic therapy on mortality in early breast cancer. An overview of 61 randomized trials among 28 896 women

Early Breast Cancer Trialists' Collaborative Group

R. Peto – presented by J. Lewis

ABSTRACT

We sought information world-wide on mortality according to assigned treatment in all randomized trials that began before 1985 of adjuvant tamoxifen or cytotoxic therapy for early breast cancer (with or without regional lymph node involvement). Coverage was reasonably complete for most countries. In 28 trials of tamoxifen nearly 4000 of 16 513 women had died, and in 40 chemotherapy trials slightly more than 4000 of 13 442 women had died. The 8106 deaths were approximately evenly distributed over years 1, 2, 3, 4 and 5+ of follow-up, with little useful information beyond year 5.

Systematic overviews of the results of these trials demonstrated reductions in mortality due to treatment that were significant when tamoxifen was compared with no tamoxifen ($p = < 0.0001$), any chemotherapy with no chemotherapy ($p = 0.003$), and polychemotherapy with single-agent chemotherapy ($p = 0.001$). In tamoxifen trials, there was a clear reduction in mortality only among women aged 50 or older, for whom assignment to tamoxifen reduced the annual odds of death during the first 5 years by about one fifth. In chemotherapy trials there was a clear reduction only among women under 50, for whom assignment to polychemotherapy reduced the annual odds of death during the first 5 years by about one quarter. Direct comparisons showed that combination chemotherapy was significantly more effective than single-agent therapy, but suggested that administration of chemotherapy for 8–24 months may offer no survival advantage over administration of the same chemotherapy for 4–6 months.

Because it involved several thousand women, this overwiew was able to demonstrate particularly clearly that both tamoxifen and cytotoxic therapy can reduce 5-year mortality.

[Adapted with permission from *N. Engl. J. Med.*, 1988, **319**, 1681–92]

8

The relationship between age and the effect of adjuvant therapies in women with primary breast cancer

A. Howell

INTRODUCTION

Apparent differences in the effectiveness of adjuvant therapies according to age have led to controversy concerning the optimum treatment for women above and below 50. In this chapter the data upon which the controversy is based and the possible reasons why chemotherapy appears more active in young women and endocrine therapy appears more active in older women will be examined.

TRIALS OF ADJUVANT THERAPY

Realization of the need to control micrometastases at the time of primary surgery in order to improve survival in patients with breast cancer led to the introduction of adjuvant systemic therapy over 40 years ago[1]. Early trials tested the effectiveness of surgical or radiotherapy-induced ovarian ablation[1]. These were followed by trials of perioperative chemotherapy[2] and later by trials of prolonged single-agent[3] and multiple-agent chemotherapy[4]. The effects of adjuvant endocrine therapy in postmenopausal women began to be tested after 1975[5].

The early results of studies using prolonged chemotherapy such as the National Surgical Adjuvant Breast and Bowel Project melphalan trial and the Milan cyclophosphamide + methotrexate + 5-fluorouracil (CMF) trial showed prolongation of disease-free survival and, after longer periods of follow-up, prolongation of survival[6, 7]. The overall survival advantages were not statistically significant; however, if the small differences detected were real they would be important considering the large number of women who develop breast cancer. In order to circumvent the problem of relatively small numbers in individual trials the results of all randomized trials of adjuvant tamoxifen or cytotoxic therapy were analysed together in an overview (Early Breast Cancer Trialists Collaborative Group 1988)[8]. This overview analysis of all trials demonstrated highly significant mortality reductions for adjuvant treatment with tamoxifen ($p < 0.0001$) and chemotherapy ($p = 0.003$) compared with controls. Tamoxifen reduced mortality by one fifth in women of 50 or more years but not for those under this age. Chemotherapy reduced mortality by one quarter in women under 50 years but there was no significant effect in women over this age. Examination of the results of treatment of women with advanced breast cancer shows that endocrine therapy and chemotherapy are active in all age groups; the purpose of this paper is to ask why there is a marked age effect when the same treatments are given as an adjuvant to surgery.

EVIDENCE FOR AN AGE EFFECT

Chemotherapy trials

In the overview analysis 7262 women were randomized into trials where various combinations of chemotherapy were compared with no adjuvant treatment (Table 1). The reduction in the annual odds of death for women < 50 was $26 \pm 7\%$ ($\pm$ SD; $n = 2526$) and for those of 50+ was $8 \pm 6\%$ ($\pm$SD; $n = 4636$). This confirms the highly significant beneficial effect of chemotherapy in younger women found in most of the individuals trials. Examination of the various types of combination chemotherapy suggested that classical CMF, as first used as an adjuvant by Bonnadonna and his co-workers[4], was the most effective regimen. The reduction in the annual odds of death in women treated with CMF was $37 \pm 7\%$ ($n = 1189$) in those < 50 and $9 \pm 9\%$ in those 50+. Examination of the effect on mortality of other types of chemotherapy shows a 12–20% reduction in the odds of death but this was not statistically significant

Table 1 Percentage reduction in the annual odds of death (± SD): chemotherapy

Chemotherapy	Age < 50	n	Age 50+	n
Single agent vs. nil	11 ± 10	(1048)	− 4 ± 10	(1209)
Multiple agents vs. nil	26 ± 7	(2526)	8 ± 6	(4636)
All CMF vs. nil	37 ± 9	(1189)	9 ± 9	(2171)
CMF + other vs. nil	20 ± 17	(450)	9 ± 13	(1027)
Other multiple vs. nil	12 ± 13	(897)	5 ± 10	(1418)

Table 2 Percentage reduction in the annual odds of recurrence and death (± SD): CMF versus nil

Age	Treated	Controls	Recurrence	Mortality
< 40	75/291	120/303	44 ± 11	46 ± 12
40–49	148/646	190/687	30 ± 8	21 ± 11
50–59	166/648	200/724	30 ± 8	7 ± 11
60+	127/501	146/538	23 ± 10	17 ± 12

(Table 1). Examination of the CMF data divided into age bands indicates that the greatest effect is seen in women < 40 and that the reductions at other ages are not significant. However, reduction in the rate of recurrence is significant in all age groups but is not converted into a significant survival advantage except for the youngest group (Table 2)[9].

Endocrine therapy

The overview analysis showed a highly significant reduction in the annual odds of death in women over 50 years of age treated with tamoxifen compared with untreated controls (19 ± 4%; $n = 9061$). There appeared to be no effect of tamoxifen in women < 50 (−1 ± 8%). This latter group consisted of comparisons of tamoxifen versus no treatment ($n = 1062$) and a larger group of patients in trials of chemotherapy and tamoxifen versus chemotherapy alone ($n = 2590$; Table 3). The reduction in the odds of death in the tamoxifen alone trials was 21 ± 14%, but −9 ± 9% when

Table 3 Percentage reduction in the annual odds of death (± SD): endocrine therapy

Treatment	Age < 50	n	Age 50+	n
Tamoxifen	21 ± 14	(1062)	19 ± 4	(9061)
Chemotherapy + tamoxifen vs.				
chemotherapy	−9 ± 9	(2590)	22 ± 6	(3800)
Ovarian ablation	19 ± 12	(1292)	10 ± 10	(1022)

chemotherapy was also used with tamoxifen. The argument for including the latter group in the overview was that the only difference in treatment was tamoxifen. However, chemotherapy causes ovarian ablation in the majority of premenopausal patients treated and is thus also an endocrine treatment itself; tamoxifen may not be expected to add to this form of indirect endocrine therapy since most trials indicate that combinations of endocrine therapies are rarely better than single therapies. Thus the conclusion of the overview analysis that tamoxifen is ineffective in women under 50 may be erroneous. When all the trials of ovarian ablation are combined the reduction in the odds of death is 19 ± 12% and is similar to the effect of tamoxifen[9]. This effect is compatible with the similarity in effect between ovarian ablation and tamoxifen in premenopausal women with advanced breast cancer[10]. However, the 95% confidence limits on the effect of these two therapies used as an adjuvant in young women include zero and further studies are required to be certain of their estimated effectiveness. It is of interest that individual trials such as the NATO and Scottish adjuvant tamoxifen trials and others show a statistically significant effect of tamoxifen in premenopausal women similar to that seen in postmenopausal women[9,11–13].

Why is chemotherapy more effective in younger women?

Given that CMF is probably the most active adjuvant chemotherapy regimen there are sufficient numbers of patients randomized in studies of this combination to be reasonably certain that treatment with it improves survival in women < 50 (Table 2). There is an effect in older women since it significantly prolongs relapse-free survival (RFS) but this is not converted into a significant survival advantage[9]. There are several possible reasons why adjuvant chemotherapy should be more active in younger women:

(1) Malignant mammary epithelial cells may be biologically different in the young;

(2) Young women tolerate treatment better and we are simply seeing a dose effect;

(3) Chemotherapy induces amenorrhoea and this may result in an indirect endocrine-mediated effect not seen in postmenopausal women;

(4) Bias against chemotherapy may be introduced because more deaths from causes other than breast cancer occur in older women; and,

(5) The effect may be due to a combination of two, three or four of the above factors.

Biological variables in relation to age

Variation in the distribution of biological characteristics of the tumour with age may account for differences in their chemosensitivity. An estimate of the possible differences is shown in Table 4. Tumours in young women tend to have fewer oestrogen and more epidermal growth factor receptors (EGFR), a higher labelling index (LI) and poorer histological grade and are more likely to be associated with a family history of breast cancer.

Hormone receptors

Most studies of the relationship between oestrogen receptor (ER) concentrations and age show an increased level with advancing years[14]. Clarke *et al.* demonstrated that this was a specific age effect rather than related to the menopause[14]. However, no correlation has been found between progesterone receptors (PR) and age[15].

First reports suggested that in patients with advanced breast cancer ER-negative tumours were more likely to respond to chemotherapy[16]. However, overview of all trials where this relationship was examined suggests that ER-positive and ER-negative tumours are equally

Table 4 Biological differences between tumours in young and old women

	Age (yr)	
	< 50	≥ 50
Oestrogen receptor	+	++
Progesterone receptor	+	+
Epidermal growth factor receptor	++	+
Labelling index	++	+
S phase fraction	+	+
DNA ploidy	+	+
Poor histological grade	++	+
Oncogene expression	+	+
Familiality	++	+

responsive[17]. Thus by inference higher proportions of patients with ER-negative tumours in the young may not account for the greater effect of adjuvant chemotherapy in this group. Although more EGFR are found in tumours from the young there are no data concerning their relationship to response to chemotherapy.

Proliferative indices

Several[18-21], but not all[22,23], studies have shown a higher LI and higher S phase fraction (demonstrated using flow cytometry) in tumours from young patients. A high LI and high S phase fraction is often associated with a poor prognosis. However, there are no unequivocal data which indicate that high LI tumours are more responsive to chemotherapy although this might be expected. Indirect evidence was reported by the Milan group[24]. In patients treated with CMF there was no difference in prognosis in patients with tumours with LI above or below the median value. In controls a difference would be expected and a lack of difference in treated patients suggests that CMF may be preferentially affecting high LI tumours and changing the prognosis to that seen with low LI tumours. There is one report which suggests that response to adjuvant therapy is unrelated to the S phase fraction[21]. Thus the data concerning proliferation and response are either equivocal or not available and further studies are required.

Tumour grade and DNA ploidy

Grading of breast cancer is based on an estimate of nuclear pleomorphism, mitotic rate and tubule formation and is thought to give an indication of tumour 'differentiation'. Early reports and more recent studies (summarized in reference 25) have demonstrated that younger patients are more likely to have histological grade III tumours with a poor nuclear grade (grade 1).

Fisher *et al.*[26] and Brinckner *et al.*[27] have demonstrated that chemotherapy with melphalan and CMF respectively is more effective in women with poorly differentiated tumours compared with well differentiated ones. Fisher noted that melphalan was only effective in poor grade tumours. When this was taken into account melphalan was active in pre- and postmenopausal women. He states that the apparent ineffectiveness of melphalan in women ≥ 50 is because there are relatively fewer poor grade tumours in this group[26]. The estimation of DNA ploidy by static or flow cytometry appears to be unrelated to age[20,23] or response to adjuvant chemotherapy[21].

Oncogene expression

Amplification of *neu* or increased expression of *ras* of loss of an allele does not appear to be correlated with age[28–30]. Data are required concerning the relationship between oncogene expression and response to adjuvant therapy.

DOSE OF CHEMOTHERAPY AND AGE

The Milan group retrospectively analysed the relationship between dose and effect of adjuvant CMF[31]. Doses were more frequently reduced in postmenopausal women; only 11% of whom received 85% or more of the scheduled dose compared with 22% of premenopausal women. This difference in dose could account for the age effect of adjuvant chemotherapy. However, this depends upon there being strong evidence for a dose–response effect with the relatively narrow range of doses used for CMF regimens. Randomized studies comparing doses are not available; there appears to be little difference in the overall effectiveness of CMF chemotherapy between groups who have used high or low doses. Strong arguments against a dose effect have recently been put forward by Henderson[32,33].

INDIRECT ENDOCRINE EFFECT OF CHEMOTHERAPY IN PREMENOPAUSAL WOMEN

Ovarian ablation results in regression in one third of patients with advanced breast cancer and improves survival when used as an adjuvant in some studies[1,34,35]. Approximately 70% of women become permanently amenorrhoeic when treated with CMF and it would be surprising if this did not cause an indirect endocrine effect of chemotherapy in some patients. This effect would be expected in patients who develop CMF-induced amenorrhoea and who are steroid hormone receptor positive. Several groups have examined their data retrospectively in order to address this question.

In the Guy's/Manchester study disease-free survival (DFS) and overall survival (OS) were associated with CMF-induced amenorrhoea and steroid hormone receptors[36]. Subsequent review showed that there was a relatively poor association with ER but a highly significant one with PR[37]. Women who developed amenorrhoea or who had PR-positive tumours had a greater DFS and OS. An effect of CMF in ER-negative tumours was in part related to the ER-negative, PR-positive subgroup which had a significantly improved survival when treated.

Five of eight studies show a longer RFS and three of four a longer OS in patients who developed CMF-induced amenorrhoea[7,27,36–40]. A longer RFS and OS was seen in patients with receptor-positive tumours in six of seven and three of four reports respectively (Table 5)[27,36–41].

The Danish study[27] is particularly important with respect to the interpretation of these results. In this study cyclophosphamide (C) alone and CMF were compared with no adjuvant therapy. The effectiveness of C with respect to RFS and OS was seen only in women with ER-positive tumours. CMF appeared equally effective in patients with ER-positive or ER-negative tumours. These data suggest that less aggressive chemotherapy is active via induced amenorrhoea whereas more aggressive therapy is associated with an additional direct cytotoxic effect.

Table 5 Effect of chemotherapy in relation to induced amenorrhoea and steroid receptors

Trial*		Amenorrhoea	Receptors
Relapse-free survival			
Milan	CMF	NS†	—
Guy's/Manchester	CMF	+	+(PR)
Denmark	C	+	+(ER)
	CMF	NS	NS(ER)
Nijmegen	CMF	+	+(PR)
Ludwig	CMF±p	+	+(ER)
ECOG	CMF±p	+	+(ER)
West Midlands	CMFVA	—	+(PR)
Survival			
Milan	CMF	NS	—
Guy's/Manchester	CMF	+	+(PR)
Nijmegen	CMF	+	+(PR)
ECOG	CMF±p	+	+(PR)
West Midlands	CMFVA	—	NS(PR)

*CMF±p, CMF±prednisone; CMFVA, CMF+vincristine+adriamycin
†NS = not significant; + = effect; — = not reported; ER = oestrogen receptor; PR = progesterone receptor

This supposition is supported by the relationship of this group's results to histological grade. C and CMF were equally effective in grade II tumours. In grade III tumours, CMF was more effective than C which in turn was more effective than control. Since grade III tumours are less likely to be receptor positive the additional effect of CMF is presumably a direct cytotoxic effect. Neither treatment was effective in grade I tumours. The suggestion that the effect of less aggressive chemotherapy is mainly mediated by an indirect endocrine effect is supported by an analysis of the Ludwig trial; in a multivariate analysis the positive effect of amenorrhoea on prognosis (RFS) was seen only in younger premenopausal patients with ER-positive tumours who received a protocol dose of CMF of 80% or less[39]. It is of interest, in this respect, that the Guy's/Manchester CMF protocol aimed to deliver 80% of the Milan dose.

COMPETING CAUSES OF DEATH IN OLDER WOMAN

Zelen and Gerber have pointed out the problems of deaths from causes other than breast cancer in the assessment of clinical trials[42]. More women die from competing causes as age increases. For example, they estimate that 10 years after primary surgery for node-positive disease the ratio of cancer deaths to other deaths would be 83.3 for women aged 40–44 but 3.7 for women aged 65–69. Although all deaths must be recorded in clinical trials this confounds the interpretation of the results in older women, for non-cancer deaths 'dilute' the apparent effectiveness of chemotherapy by reducing the statistical efficiency of trials. A larger number of older patients are required to be certain of the differences found and, because of the size of most of our trials, they may lead to an underestimation of the effect of chemotherapy in this group (for details see reference 42). However, this problem has not prevented the demonstration of a highly significant positive effect of tamoxifen in older women and such problems must be circumvented to some extent by overview analyses[8].

COMBINATIONS OF THE ABOVE FACTORS

It is likely that no single factor is responsible for the observation that chemotherapy is apparently more active in young women. The data appear to point mainly in two directions. Some studies suggest that tumour characteristics are important and others that chemotherapy-induced ovarian ablation is important. It is probable that both chemotherapy-induced amenorrhoea and biological differences in the tumours of the young are important. From a patient's viewpoint we need to know the magnitude of the additional direct cytotoxic effect of chemotherapy. A small effect may not be worth the additional toxicity, a large effect would.

IMPLICATION FOR FUTURE STUDIES

It is unlikely that the results of adjuvant therapy can be improved using the conventional treatments we have available. The immediate goal of oncologists should be to deliver appropriate available treatments with the minimum possible toxicity. Advances will probably be made by the use of high intensity chemotherapy with haemopoetic growth factors and the development of new types of endocrine therapy based on growing knowledge of local growth factors in the control of epithelial cell proliferation. Until new treatments have been developed it is appropriate to pursue trials which will refine our knowledge of the appropriate treatments to use in particular groups of patients.

Data from the overview of trials of ovarian ablation and tamoxifen in premenopausal women suggest that endocrine therapy is active in this group[8]. In the National Cancer Institute consensus meeting the ovarian ablation data were not presented and it was concluded that tamoxifen was ineffective in young women. There is a high probability that this conclusion was erroneous and that endocrine therapy is effective particularly in women between the ages of 40 and 49. For example in this group the overview analysis showed that CMF resulted in a $21 \pm 11\%$ reduction in the annual odds of death; whereas when tamoxifen was used alone there was a $21 \pm 14\%$ reduction in the annual odds of death. However, it is hard to believe that endocrine therapy could match the improvement of $46 \pm 12\%$ in OS seen with CMF chemotherapy in women less than 40 years of age. Trials of ovarian ablation with or without tamoxifen compared with standard CMF in premenopausal women of 40+ would appear to be a logical approach to assessing the magnitude and value of any additional cytotoxic effect of CMF above its indirect endocrine effect.

A preliminary report of such a trial was presented at the 1988 St Gallen meeting[43]. One hundred and nineteen patients with one to three positive nodes were randomized to receive tamoxifen 30 mg daily or CMF at conventional doses. CMF was superior for RFS ($p = 0.08$) and OS ($p = 0.002$). A trial of ovarian ablation versus CMF is in progress in Scotland but the results are not yet available. The Danish study[27] of nil versus C versus CMF showed that for grade II tumours C (which appeared to act via an endocrine mechanism) was equivalent to CMF. CMF may have an additional effect in grade III tumours and it is the magnitude of this which we need to know.

CONCLUSIONS

(1) It is probable that all women <40 should be offered classical CMF adjuvant therapy.

(2) There is doubt concerning the relative value of CMF and endocrine therapy in women of 40–49. Trials comparing these approaches or of adding chemotherapy to endocrine therapy versus endocrine therapy alone are indicated.

(3) Such studies would need to be large and should therefore include many centres.

(4) Data concerning grade (and its components), LI and S phase fraction and ER, PR and EGFR measurements on all tumours should be collected. This would entail quality control measures between centres in order to standardize assays or a central reference laboratory.

REFERENCES

1. Cole, M.P. (1970). Prophylactic compared with therapeutic X-ray artificial menopause. In Joslin, C.A.F. and Gleave, E.N. (eds.) *The Clinical Management of Advanced Breast Cancer*, 2nd Tenovus Workshop, pp. 2–11. (Cardiff: Alpha Omega Alpha Publishing)

2. Fisher, B., Slack, N., Katrych, D. *et al.* (1975). Ten-year follow up results of patients with carcinoma of the breast in a cooperative clinical trial evaluating surgical adjuvant chemotherapy. *Surg. Gynecol. Obstet.*, **140**, 528–34

3. Koyama, H., Wada, T., Takahashi, Y. *et al.* (1980). Surgical adjuvant chemotherapy with mitomycin C and cyclophosphamide in Japanese patients with breast cancer. *Cancer*, **46**, 2373–9

4. Bonadonna, G., Valagussa, P., Rossi, A. *et al.* (1985). Ten-year experience with CMF-based adjuvant chemotherapy in resectable breast cancer. *Breast Cancer Res. Treat.*, **5**, 95–115

5. Palshof, T., Mouridsen, H.T. and Daehnfeldt, J.L. (1980). Adjuvant endocrine therapy of breast cancer. A controlled clinical trial of oestrogen and anti-oestrogen: preliminary results of the Copenhagen breast cancer trials. In Henningsen, B., Linder, F. and Steichele, C. (eds.) *Endocrine Treatment of Breast Cancer, A New Approach*, pp. 185–9. (New York: Springer-Verlag)

6. Fisher, B. Fisher, E.R., Redmond, C. and participating NSABP investigators (1986). Ten year results from the National Surgical Adjuvant Breast and Bowel Project (NSABP) clinical trial evaluating the use of L-Phenylalanine mustard (L-PAM) in the management of primary breast cancer. *J. Clin. Oncol.*, **4**, 929–41

7. Bonadonna, G., Valagussa, P., Tancini, G. *et al.* (1980). Current status of Milan adjuvant chemotherapy trials for node-positive and node-negative breast cancer. *National Cancer Inst. Monogr.*, **1**, 45–9

8. Early Breast Cancer Trialists Collaborative Group. (1990). The effects of adjuvant tamoxifen and of cytotoxic therapy on mortality in early breast cancer. An overview of 61 randomized trials among 28,896 women. *N. Engl. J. Med.*, in press

9. Early Breast Cancer Trialists Co-operative Group. *J. Natl. Cancer Inst.*, in press

10. Buchanan, R.B., Blamey, R.W., Durrant, K.R., Howell, A., Peterson, A.G., Preece, P.E., Smith, D.C., Williams, C.J. and Wilson, R.G. (1986). A randomized comparison of tamoxifen with surgical oophorectomy in premenopausal patients with advanced breast cancer. *J. Clin. Oncol.*, **49**, 1326–30

11. (1987). Adjuvant tamoxifen in early breast cancer. NATO trial. *Lancet*, **ii**, 191–2

12. (1987). Adjuvant tamoxifen in the management of operable breast cancer: the Scottish Trial. Report from the Breast Cancer Trials Committee, The Scottish Cancer Trials Office (MRC), Edinburgh. *Lancet*, **ii**, 171–5

13. Redmond, C.K., Fisher, B., Constantino, J., Wickerham, D.L., Wolmark, N., Fisher, E. and NSABP contributing investigators. (1988). Treatment of stage I breast cancer: the NSABP experience. *Proceedings of the International Conference on Endocrine Therapy*, Monaco, Nov. 19–21, 1988

14. Clark, G.M., Osborne, C.K. and McGuire, W.L. (1984). Correlations between estrogen receptor, progesterone receptor and patient characteristics in human breast cancer. *J. Clin. Oncol.*, **2**, 1102–9

15. McGuire, W.L. and Clark, G.M. (1983). The prognostic role of progesterone receptors in human breast cancer. *Sem. Oncol.*, **10**, 2–6

16. Lippman, M.E., Allegra, J.C., Thompson, E.B., Simon, R., Barlock, A., Green, L., Huff, K.K., Huff, H.M.T., Airken, S.C. and Warren, R. (1978). The relation between estrogen receptors and response rate of cytotoxic chemotherapy in metastatic breast cancer. *N. Engl. J. Med.*, **298**, 1223

17. Rubens, R.D. (1981). Breast cancer. In Pinedo, H.M. (ed.) *Cancer Chemotherapy*, pp. 360–96

18. Meyer, J.S. (1986). Cell kinetics in selection and stratification of patients for adjuvant therapy of breast carcinoma. *Natl. Cancer Inst. Monogr.*, **1**, 25–34

19. Silvestrini, R., Daidone, M.G. and Di Fronzo, G. (1979). Relationship between proliferative activity and estrogen receptors in breast cancer. *Cancer*, **44**, 665–70

20. Dressler, L.G., Seamer, L.C., Owens, M.A., Clark, G.M. and McGuire, W.L. (1988). DNA flow cytometry and prognostic factors in 1331 frozen breast cancer specimens. *Cancer*, **61**, 420–7

21. Hedley, D.W., Rugg, C.A. and Gelber, R.D. (1987). Association of DNA index and S-phase fraction with prognosis of nodes positive early breast cancer. *Cancer Res.*, **47**, 4729–35

22. Héry, M., Gioanni, J., Lalanne, C.M., Namer, M. and Courdie, A. (1987). The DNA labelling index: a prognostic factor in node negative breast cancer. *Br. Cancer Res. Treat.*, **9**, 207–11

23. Feichter, G.E., Mueller, A., Kaufmann, M., Haag, D., Born, J.A., Abel, U. and Klinga, K. (1988). Correlation of DNA flow cytometric results and other prognostic factors in primary breast cancer. *Int. J. Cancer*, **41**, 823–8

24. Daidone, M.G., Silvestrini, R., Canova, S., Orefice, S. and Bonadonna, G. (1987). Cell kinetics and prognosis in human breast cancer. *4th EORTC Breast Cancer Working Conference 1987*, Abstract no.D4.6.

25. Stoll, B.A. Components of a prognostic index. In Stoll, B.A. (ed.) *Breast Cancer Treatment and Prognosis*, pp. 115–31. (Oxford: Blackwell)

26. Fisher, E.R., Redmond, C. and Fisher, B. (1983). Pathologic findings from the National Surgical Adjuvant Breast Project VII. Relationship of chemotherapeutic responsiveness to tumour differentiation. *Cancer*, **51**, 181

27. Brinckner, H., Rose, C., Rank, F., Mouridsen, H.T., Jakobsen, A., Dombernowsky, P., Panduro, J. and Anderson, K.W. (1987). Evidence of a castration-mediated effect of adjuvant cytotoxic chemotherapy in premenopausal breast cancer. *J. Clin. Oncol.*, **5**, 1771–8

28. Salmon, D.J., Clark, G.M, Wong, S.G., Levin, W.J., Ullrich, A. and McGuire, W.L. (1987). Human breast cancer: correlation of relapse and survival with amplification of the HER-2/neu oncogene. *Science*, **235**, 177–82

29. Agnantis, N.J., Parissi, P., Anagnostakis, D. and Spandidos, D. (1986). A comparative study of Harvey-ras oncogene expression with conventional clinicopathologic parameters of breast cancer. *Oncology*, **43**, 36–9

30. Theillet, C., Lidereau, R., Escot, C., Hutzell, P., Brunet, M., Gest, J., Schlom, J. and Callahan, R. (1986). Loss of a c-H-ras 1 allele and aggressive human primary breast carcinomas. *Cancer Res.*, **46**, 4776–81

31. Bonadonna, G. and Valagussa, P. (1981). Dose response effect of adjuvant chemotherapy in breast cancer. *N. Engl. J. Med.*, **304**, 10–15

32. Henderson, I.C. (1987). Adjuvant systemic therapy for early breast cancer. *Curr. Probl. Cancer*, **11**, 123–207

33. Henderson, I.C., Hayes, D.F. and Gelman, R. (1988). Dose-response in the treatment of breast cancer. A critical review. *J. Clin. Oncol.*, **6**, 1501–16

34. Meakin, J.W., Allt, W.E.C., Beale, F.A., Bush, R.S., Clark, R.M., Fitzpatrick, P.J., Hawkins, N.V., Jenkin, R.D.T., Pringle, J.F., Reid, J.G., Rider, W.D., Hayward, J.L. and Bulbrook, R.D. (1988). Ovarian irradiation and prednisone following surgery and radiotherapy for carcinoma of the breast. *Breast Cancer Res. Treat.*, **3**, 45–8

35. Bryant, A.J. and Weir, J.A. (1981). Prophylactic oophorectomy in operable instances of carcinoma of the breast. *Surg. Gynecol. Obstet.*, **153**, 660–4

36. Howell, A., Bush, H., George, W.D. *et al.* (1984). Controlled trial of adjuvant chemotherapy with cyclophosphamide, methotrexate, and fluorouracil for breast cancer. *Lancet*, **ii**, 307–11

37. Padmanabhan, N., Howell, A. and Rubens, R.D. (1986). Mechanism of action of adjuvant chemotherapy in early breast cancer. *Lancet*, **ii**, 411–14

38. Beex, L.V.A.M., Mackenzie, M.A., Raemaekers, J.M.M., Smals, A.G.H., Benraad, Th.J. and Kloppenborg, P.W.C. (1988). Adjuvant chemotherapy in premenopausal patients with primary breast cancer; relation to drug-induced amenorrhoea, age and the progesterone receptor status of the tumour. *Eur. J. Cancer Clin. Oncol.*, **24**, 719–21

39. Ludwig Breast Cancer Study Group. (1985). Randomized trial of adjuvant combination chemotherapy with or without prednisone in premenopausal breast cancer patients with metastases in one to three axillary lymph nodes. *Cancer Res.*, **45**, 4454–9

40. Tormey, D.C. (1984). Adjuvant systemic therapy in postoperative node-positive patients with breast carcinoma: The CALB trial and the ECOG premenopausal trial. *Recent Results in Cancer Research. Adjuvant Chemotherapy of Breast Cancer*, pp. 155–65. (Heidelberg: Springer-Verlag)

41. Morrison, J.M., Howell, A., Grieve, R.J. *et al.* (1984). The West Midlands Oncology Association trials of adjuvant chemotherapy for operable breast cancer. In Jones, S.E. and Salmon, S.E. (eds.) *Adjuvant Therapy of Cancer IV*, pp. 253–9. (Orlando: Grune & Stratton)

42. Zelen, M. and Gelman, R. (1986). Assessment of adjuvant trials in breast cancer. *Natl. Cancer Inst. Monogr.*, **1**, 11–17

43. Kaufmann, M. (1988). Treatment results with endocrine, chemo and chemo-hormono-therapy in premenopausal patients. *Adjuvant Therapy of Primary Breast Cancer. 3rd International Conference*, St Gallen/Switzerland, March 2–5, 1988

9

Pharmacology of the luteinizing hormone releasing hormone (LHRH) analogue, Zoladex*

B.J.A. Furr

INTRODUCTION

It is well established that androgens stimulate the growth of a majority of prostate cancers, and oestrogens enhance the growth of many breast cancers. A variety of approaches has been adopted to induce androgen or oestrogen withdrawal from the tumour cell in order to prevent prostate and breast tumour progression. Antioestrogens such as Nolvadex[1*] and antiandrogens such as cyproterone acetate[2], flutamide[3], nilutamide[4] and Casodex[5*], compete with the relevant stimulatory hormone to bind to a cytosolic receptor protein, but have little or no intrinsic activity as oestrogens or androgens, respectively.

A knowledge of the processes that regulate gonadal steroid synthesis has led to further approaches to tumour therapy. Administration of oestrogens to men with prostate cancer inhibits gonadotropin secretion from the pituitary gland, leading to a form of medical castration[6]. However, the clinical benefits seen in prostate cancer patients may be counterbalanced by serious cardiovascular complications[7].

*Zoladex, Nolvadex and Casodex are trade names, the property of Imperial Chemical Industries PLC

89

Recently, the availability of potent analogues of luteinizing hormone releasing hormone (LHRH) has led to a selective effect on pituitary gonadotropin release that produces a form of medical castration. The side-effects are markedly less than those associated with the administration of oestrogens and indeed the only side-effects reported are those which might be predicted from a medical castration. Zoladex (goserelin, D-Ser (Bu^t)^6, Azgly^{10}-LHRH; Figure 1), is a potent LHRH analogue, which can be used for the treatment of hormone-responsive disease[8]. This paper describes pharmacological studies with Zoladex, attempts to explain its mode of action and reports on an innovative depot formulation which allows the drug to be released continuously over at least 28 days.

Pyro - Glu - His - Trp - Ser - Tyr - Gly - Leu - Arg - Pro - Gly - NH$_2$

LH - RH

Pyro - Glu - His - Trp - Ser - Tyr - |D - Ser (Bu^t)| - Leu - Arg - Pro - |Azgly NH$_2$|

ZOLADEX (ICI 118,630 D - SER (Bu ^{t})^6 AzGly^{10} - LH - RH)

Figure 1   Structures of LHRH and Zoladex

PHARMACOLOGICAL STUDIES WITH AQUEOUS SOLUTIONS OF AN LHRH AGONIST – ZOLADEX

Zoladex is an LHRH agonist and when given acutely, will induce secretion of follicle stimulating hormone (FSH) and luteinizing hormone (LH). In the rat, a single intramuscular injection of 5 µg Zoladex elicits a supraphysiological release of LH (Figure 2). In this respect it is at least 100 times as potent as LHRH[9].

Zoladex will also initiate LH release and ovulation in androgen-sterilized constant-oestrus rats (Table 1). When given by the intramuscular (i.m.), subcutaneous (s.c.) or intravenous (i.v.), routes, Zoladex is at least 100 times as potent as LHRH. It should be emphasized, however, that it is far less effective when given intravaginally, orally (p.o.) or intranasally, and in the latter case absorption is both low and variable.

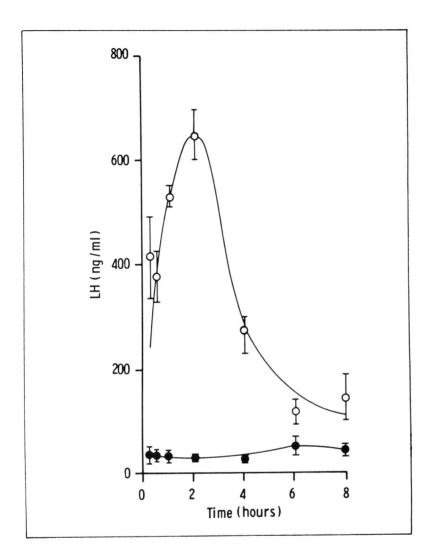

Figure 2 Plasma LH concentrations in mature virgin female rats given a single i.m. injection of 5 μg Zoladex at time 0 (open circles). The closed circles are the values for saline-treated controls. The points indicated are the mean values ± SEM for five animals

Table 1 Induction of ovulation with Zoladex given intravenously, orally, intravaginally or intranasally in androgen-sterilized, constant-oestrus rats

Route	Dose (μg)	Number ovulating/ number treated	Response (%)
Intravenous	0.005	9/9	100
	0.0031	10/18	55.6
	0.0016	5/21	23.8
	0.0008	0/12	0
Oral	25	3/3	100
	10	5/6	83.3
	5	5/12	41.7
	2.5	2/6	33
Intravaginal	25	2/3	67
	10	0/3	0
Intranasal	1	2/5	40

The high potency of Zoladex is partly due to its enhanced affinity for the pituitary LHRH receptor (Figure 3), which leads to around a 10-fold greater potency compared with LHRH, in releasing LH from pituitary cells in culture (Figure 4). The high potency *in vivo* is also due to a longer elimination half-life: in man, the half-life of Zoladex is more than 4 h, compared with less than 10 min for LHRH[10].

When given chronically, Zoladex induces inhibition of gonadal steroid secretion and produces a castration-like state in rats, dogs and primates[8,11,12]. At first sight, this is unexpected and has therefore been inappropriately described as the paradoxical effect of LHRH agonists. An explanation for this observation is clearly required.

MODE OF ACTION OF LHRH AGONISTS

Normally, LHRH is released from the hypothalamus as a series of small pulses, at approximately 90-min intervals[13,14]. The LHRH travels via the hypothalamic–pituitary portal system to the pituitary gland where it binds to LHRH receptors present on the cell surface. Receptors occupied

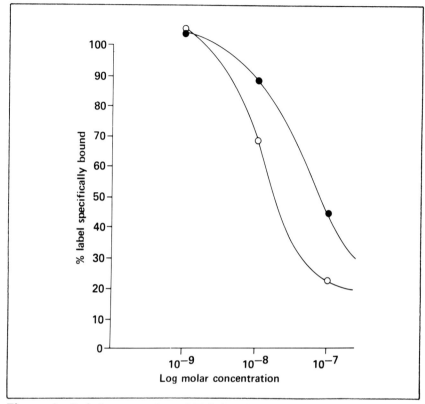

Figure 3 Relative potencies of Zoladex (O) and LHRH (●) in causing displacement of [^{125}I]D-Leu^6-proethylamide^9-LHRH from a rat pituitary membrane receptor preparation

by LHRH aggregate into clumps, 'coated pits' are formed and the receptor–ligand complex is internalized, thus disappearing from the cell surface. There is usually an excess of LHRH receptors present on the pituitary cell and receptor resynthesis occurs. This process allows an orderly and systematic secretion of LH. When an LHRH agonist is first given at a relatively high dosage, the majority of LHRH receptors are occupied and subsequently internalized. This leads to supraphysiological LH secretion and an intitial stimulation of gonadal function. However, the marked loss of LH receptors and the failure of receptor replenishment due to the continuing presence of LHRH agonists leads to a pituitary cell which has few receptors, and is, therefore, unable to respond to LHRH agonists. Consequently, LH secretion is markedly reduced, resulting in

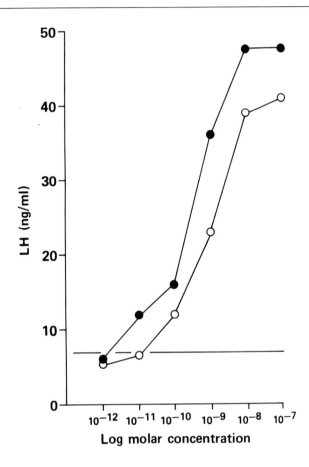

Figure 4 Release of LH from dispersed rat pituitary cells into the culture medium after 4 h incubation in response to increasing concentrations of Zoladex (●) and LHRH (O). Control values shown by the horizontal line indicate the release rate in the absence of LHRH or LHRH agonist

gonadal atrophy, a reduction in steroid secretion and the regression of hormone-responsive tissues including mammary and prostate tumours.

This phenomenon had long been recognized and termed either tachyphylaxis or tissue desensitization, but is now described as receptor down-regulation. It is clearly a predictable, non-paradoxical effect of chronic therapy with LHRH agonists. Usually tachyphylaxis is regarded as a serious disadvantage in drug therapy. Here, for the first time, advantage is taken of this phenomenon to produce an effective therapy.

DEVELOPMENT AND PROPERTIES OF A DEPOT FORMULATION OF ZOLADEX

Although early preclinical studies clearly demonstrate the effectiveness of daily s.c. injections of Zoladex in inducing regression of sex hormone-responsive tumours[11], it was felt that this would limit clinical acceptability and reduce patient compliance with therapy. Several formulations were considered, but the majority were rejected because of concerns about reliability of drug delivery or convenience. Administration of Zoladex by vaginal pessaries limited treatment to women, and absorption was low and variable. Similarly, in our experience, absorption of the drug after nasal administration was also low and unacceptably variable. Furthermore, nasal application had to be made several times daily to achieve the desired biological effect, which again raised concerns about the likelihood of compliance. Others have found nasal spray formulations to be acceptable, but compliance is recognized as a problem[15].

The target selected for a drug delivery system for Zoladex was the development of a biodegradable, sustained-release formulation that would deliver the drug over a period of at least 28 days. Efforts were concentrated on poly(D,L-lactide) and poly(D,L-lactide-*co*-glycolide) since these have been used for the sustained delivery of low molecular weight compounds such as steroids[16], narcotic antagonists[17] and antimalarial drugs[18]. Moreover, since these polymers have been evaluated as biodegradable surgical sutures and prostheses, it is known that they are both pharmaceutically and toxicologically acceptable. This work culminated in the development of a depot based on a 50:50 poly(D,L-lactide-*co*-glycolide) polymer throughout which the drug is homogeneously dispersed. The depot is in the form of a rod approximately 1 mm in diameter and 3–6 mm in length containing 500–1000 µg Zoladex. Following administration of a single depot containing 500 µg Zoladex, oestrogen secretion, assessed by vaginal smear inspection, is suppressed in adult female rats for 33 days (Figure 5).

Although the primary objective was to produce a formulation of the drug that was more convenient to administer and that would secure improved compliance, the depot formulation also appears to have improved efficacy. This was demonstrated in rats that were given a single s.c. bolus dose of 50 µg Zoladex for 6 weeks or, alternatively, at the start of the experiment and at 4 weeks, a single s.c. depot, calculated to release

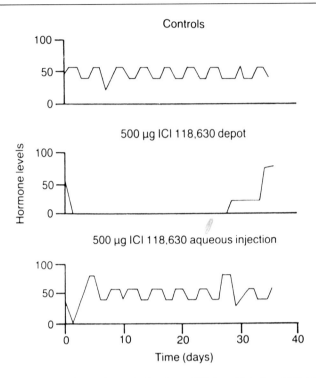

Figure 5 Effect of a single s.c. injection of 500 µg Zoladex (ICI 118,630) either as a depot formulation or as an aqueous injection in 1% hydroxymethylcellulose on ovarian activity in adult female rats. Control data are shown in the upper panel for comparison

a dose of Zoladex equivalent to 50 µg daily. Rats were killed at various times after the final treatment and serum LH was determined by radioimmunoassay in blood collected from the dorsal aorta (Figure 6).

As expected, the bolus dose of Zoladex elicited a massive secretion of LH in rats pretreated with saline. In spite of pretreatment for 6 weeks with 50 µg Zoladex daily, the bolus dose of the drug still caused a substantial release of LH, although a clear degree of desensitization of the pituitary gland occurred. In contrast, there was negligible LH secretion in response to the bolus injection in rats pretreated with Zoladex depot, indicating an improved level of pituitary desensitization by this formulation. Similarly, in the male monkey, *Maccaca nemestrina*, the depot formulation of Zoladex induces a fall in plasma testosterone into the castrate range, whereas daily s.c. injections are relatively ineffective. (It should be noted that recovery

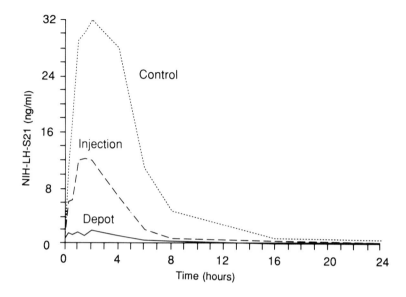

Figure 6 Effect of a 50 μg s.c. bolus dose of Zoladex on LH release in mature male rats given either saline or 50 μg Zoladex daily or a single s.c. depot containing Zoladex calculated to release approximately 50 μg daily at the start of the experiment and at day 28. The bolus dose of 50 μg Zoladex was injected 6 weeks after the start of the experiment and serum LH was measured by radioimmunoassay at the times shown

of testicular function occurred around 40 days after the final depot was administered.) This advantage of depot Zoladex has also been observed in the clinic where incomplete pituitary desensitization is seen in some patients given daily s.c. injections of the drug, in contrast to complete pituitary desensitization in those given Zoladex depot[19].

EFFECTS OF DEPOT ZOLADEX IN ANIMALS BEARING SEX HORMONE-RESPONSIVE TUMOURS

The androgen-responsive, Dunning R3327H, transplantable rat prostate tumour[20] was used in several studies to determine the efficacy of Zoladex depot administration. Single s.c. depots containing 1 mg Zoladex given every 28 days to rats bearing Dunning R3327H prostate tumours, implanted on each flank, produced a marked inhibition of tumour growth, similar to that seen in surgically castrated rats (Figure 7). Twenty-one days after the eighth depot was given, the rats were killed and the weights of the sex organs assessed and serum hormone concentrations measured by radioimmunoassay. Testes weights were about 10% of those of control rats of a similar age and weight, and showed atrophic histological changes; ventral prostate gland and seminal vesicle weights were identical to those in the surgically castrated group and, histologically, were also completely atrophic. Serum LH and testosterone were undetectable in the group given Zoladex depot and serum FSH level was decreased by 60–70%.

A comparison was made of the efficacy of surgical castration, depot Zoladex, a new peripherally-selective antiandrogen, ICI 176,334 (Casodex)[5] and the combination, in the treatment of Dunning R3327H prostate tumours (Figure 8). All treatments produced a significant

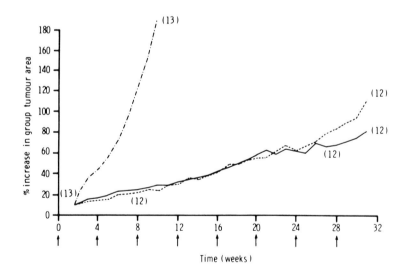

Figure 7 Growth of Dunning R3327H androgen-responsive prostate tumours in male rats which were either surgically castrated (—) or given a single s.c. depot without Zoladex (·–·–) or containing 1 mg Zoladex (----) at 28-day intervals on eight occasions as shown by the arrows. The values are expressed as percentage increase in mean tumour area

Estimated Mean Tumour Areas With Standard Errors (Geometric)

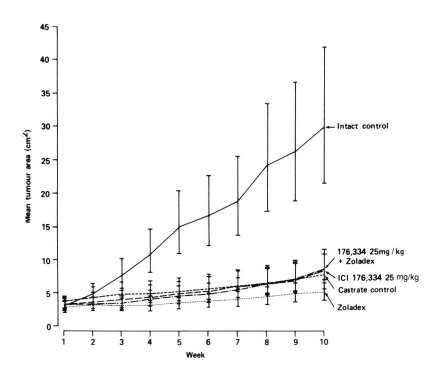

Figure 8   Effect of surgical castration, depot Zoladex given s.c. every 28 days, ICI 176,334 (novel peripherally-selective antiandrogen) given p.o. daily and the combination of the two drugs on growth of the Dunning R3327H prostate tumour. Data from intact control animals are shown for comparison. The results show the mean tumour area ± SEM

reduction in tumour growth compared to control animals, but none of the treatments was any more effective than another. Since the rat does not secrete significant quantities of adrenal androgens, these data cannot be taken to disprove the total androgen withdrawal hypothesis advanced by Labrie and colleagues[21].

Zoladex depot has also proved to be highly effective against dimethylbenzanthracene-induced rat mammary tumours. Administration of single s.c. depots containing 500 μg Zoladex every 28 days produced inhibition of oestrogen secretion, disappearance of cornified cells from vaginal smears and frequently, complete tumour regression[11]. When given at days 30, 58 and 86 after administration of the carcinogen, single depots containing 500 μg Zoladex delayed the appearance of tumours for a period of around 100 days, i.e. the expected duration of action of such a treatment regimen[11].

When given at 28-day intervals, starting on day 30 after administration of the carcinogen, single s.c. depots of Zoladex caused a more profound inhibition of tumour appearance and only nine out of 27 rats had mammary tumours at the end of the study on day 450[11]. The tumours that remained did not regress following ovariectomy, and were therefore classified as non-hormone responsive. It is concluded from this study (which approximates the adjuvant therapy setting) that Zoladex may be of benefit as a treatment for primary breast cancer after mastectomy in premenopausal women.

No side-effects were observed in any of these studies, and there was no lesion at any injection site.

CONCLUSION

Zoladex, in common with other potent LHRH agonistic analogues when given chronically at relatively high doses, causes a predictable pituitary desensitization and consequently an inhibition of pituitary gonadotropin secretion. This in turn leads to gonadal and accessory sex organ atrophy.

The biodegradable, biocompatible Zoladex depot which releases the drug continuously over at least 28 days, is both more convenient to administer and more efficacious in a number of test systems than are daily s.c. injections. In particular, it is highly effective at inducing regression of sex hormone-responsive prostate and mammary tumours. The pharmacological profile of Zoladex depot, its excellent tolerance and its convenience of administration make it an effective alternative to surgery for treatment of sex hormone-responsive tumours in men and women, and in a number of other disorders dependent upon or modified by gonadal sex steroids.

ACKNOWLEDGEMENTS

I would like to thank NIAMDD, Professor L.E. Reichert and G.D. Niswender for reagents for FSH, LH and prolactin radioimmunoassays; the US National Prostate Cancer Agency for supplies of rats bearing Dunning R3327H tumours; and the many colleagues in ICI Pharmaceuticals Research Department, who have made this development possible, particularly A.S. Dutta, F.G. Hutchinson and B.E. Valcaccia. This paper originally appeared in *Hormone Research* (1989) published by S. Karger AG, Basel.

REFERENCES

1. Furr, B.J.A. and Jordan, V.C. (1984). The pharmacology and clinical uses of tamoxifen. *Pharmacol. Ther.*, **25**, 127–205
2. Neumann, F. (1987). Pharmacology and clinical uses of cyproterone acetate. In Furr, B.J.A. and Wakeling, A.E. (eds.) *Pharmacology and Clinical Uses of Inhibitors of Hormone Secretion and Action,* pp. 132–59. (London: Balliere Tindall)
3. Neri, R. and Kassem, N. (1987). Pharmacology and clinical uses of flutamide. In Furr, B.J.A. and Wakeling, A.E. (eds.) *Pharmacology and Clinical Uses of Inhibitors of Hormone Secretion and Action,* pp. 160–9. (London: Balliere Tindall)
4. Moguilewsky, M., Fiet, J., Tournemine, G. and Raynaud, J-P. (1986). Pharmacology of an anti-androgen, Anandron, used as an adjuvant therapy in the treatment of prostate cancer. *J. Steroid Biochem.*, **24**, 139–46
5. Furr, B.J.A., Valaccia, B., Curry, B., Woodburn, J.R., Chesterson, G. and Tucker, H. (1987). ICI 176,334: a novel non-steroidal, peripherally selective anti-androgen. *J. Endocrinol.*, **113**, R7–R9
6. Robinson, M.R.G. (1982). Carcinoma of the prostate: hormonal therapy. In Furr, B.J.A. (ed.) *Clinics in Oncology*, vol. 1, pp. 233–43. (London: Saunders)
7. Veterans Administration Cooperative Urological Research Group (1967). Treatment and survival of patients with cancer of the prostate. *Surg. Gynecol. Obstet.*, **124**, 1011–17
8. Furr, B.J.A. (1987). Treatment of hormone-responsive rat mammary and prostate tumours with Zoladex depot. In Klijn, J.G.M., Paridaens, R. and Foekens, J.A. (eds.) *Hormonal Manipulation of Cancer: Peptides, Growth Factors and New (Anti) Steroidal Agents.* Monograph Series of the European Organisation for Research on Treatment of Cancer (EORTC), vol. 18, pp. 213–23. (New York: Raven Press)
9. Maynard, P.V. and Nicholson, R.I. (1979). Biological effects of high dose

levels of a series of new LHRH analogues in intact female rats. *Br. J. Cancer,* **39**, 274–9

10. Swaisland, A.J., Adam, H.K., Barker, Y., Holmes, B. and Hutchinson, F.G. (1988). Tailored release profiles for Zoladex using biodegradable polymers. *Pharm. Weekbl.,* **10**, 57

11. Furr, B.J.A. and Nicholson, R.I. (1982). Use of analogues of luteinising hormone-releasing hormone for the treatment of cancer. *J. Reprod. Fertil.,* **64**, 529–39

12. Furr, B.J.A. and Hutchinson, F.G. (1985). Biodegradable sustained release formulation of the LHRH analogue Zoladex for the treatment of hormone-responsive tumours. In Schroeder, F.H. and Richards, B. (eds.) EORTC Genitourinary Group Monograph 2, Part A. *Therapeutic Principles in Metastatic Prostatic Cancer.* Progress in Clinical and Biochemical Research, vol. 185A, pp. 143–53. (New York: Liss)

13. Nankin, H.R. and Troen, R. (1971). Repetitive luteinising hormone elevations in serum of normal men. *J. Clin. Endocrinol. Metab.,* **33**, 558–60

14. Santen, R.J. and Bardin, C.W. (1973). Episodic luteinising hormone secretion in man. *J. Clin. Invest.,* **52**, 2617–28

15. Rajfer, J., Handelsman, D.J., Crum, A., Steiner, B., Peterson, M. and Swerdloff, R.S. (1986). Comparison of the efficacy of subcutaneous and nasal spray buserelin treatment in suppression of testicular steroidogenesis in men with prostate cancer. *Fertil. Steril.,* **46**, 104–10

16. Beck, L.R., Cowsar, D.R., Lewis, D.H., Cosgrove, J.R., Riddle, C.T., Lowry, S.L. and Epperly, T. (1979). A new long-acting injectable microcapsule system for the administration of progesterone. *Fertil. Steril.,* **31**, 545–51

17. Schwope, A.D., Wise, D.L. and Howed, J.F. (1975). Lactic/glycolic acid polymers as narcotic antagonist delivery systems. *Life Sci.,* 1877–85

18. Wise, D.L., McCormick, G.J., Willet, G.P. and Anderson, L.C. (1976). Sustained release of an antimalarial drug using copolymer of glycolic/lactic acid. *Life Sci.,* 867–73

19. Grant, J.B.F., Ahmed, S.R., Shalet, S.M., Costello, C.B., Howell, A. and Blacklock, N.J. (1986). Testosterone and gonadotrophin profiles in patients on daily or monthly LHRH analogue (Zoladex) compared with orchidectomy. *Br. J. Urol.,* **58**, 539–44

20. Smolev, J.K., Heston, W.D.W., Scott, W.W. and Coffey, D.S. (1977). Characterization of the Dunning R3327H prostatic adenocarcinoma: an appropriate animal model for prostatic cancer. *Cancer Treat. Rep.,* **61**, 273–87

21. Labrie, F., Dupont, A. and Belanger, A. (1985). Complete androgen blockade for the treatment of prostate cancer. In De Vita, V.T. Jr, Hellman, S. and Rosenberg, S.A. (eds.) *Important Advances in Oncology,* pp. 193–217. (Philadelphia: Lippincott)

10

The assessment and interpretation of quality of life in patients with breast cancer

P.E. Preece

Since 1948, when Karnofsky devised his scale to measure the quality of life in patients with cancer[1], repeated attempts have been made to achieve this aim. In practice the major difficulties have been to find a method of measuring quality of life which is easy to administer, reproducible and valid statistically.

The perception of quality of life differs between individuals and probably even for single individuals at different times and under different circumstances[2]. As a result we speak of quality of life as 'subjective', and regard such as being more difficult or even impossible to measure compared with 'objective' parameters. Yet to the patient the subjective factors are usually of much more importance than the objective. For example, it matters much more to such a patient that she is anorexic than that her abdominal girth has increased 3 cm in the past 24 hours.

Thus the need to determine more accurately and more sensitively the experiences and feelings of our patients puts an onus on clinicians to assess quality of life[3]. Two other factors increase the urgency that this aim be satisfactorily achieved soon. These are respectively economical and pharmaceutical. New efficacious drugs and other treatments are steadily being promoted for the management of patients with cancer. Proper comparison between these and their comparative costs will necessitate measurement of both subjective as well as objective effects. Although equally effective in such parameters as tumour-free interval, different drugs may have different effects in regard to such sensations as appetite, libido, sense of well being, all of which need to be appraised in the overall determination of the relative merits of the agents.

Many instruments have been devised for assessing and measuring the quality of life. For some the measurement is expressed as a single aggregated score known as an 'Index' such as that of Karnofsky where the index is a percentage (Table 1). Others result in a 'Profile', which is a series of numbers, each of which quantifies a different discrete parameter. An example is the Sickness Impact Profile (SIP) which consists of 136 items grouped into 12 categories[4]. An index is less sensitive but simpler, a profile is more specific but more complex. Some instruments are designed for single use, such as in screening a particular cohort or community. In clinical practice and trials, instruments are needed which are capable of multiple repeated administration, so that changes may be observed and measured. Some instruments measure health parameters in general (e.g. SIP[4]), whereas many are disease-specific, e.g. the Arthritis Impact Measurement Scale[5] (AIMS) and the Functional Living Index for Cancer[6] (FLIC). For maximum efficiency, in addition to being disease-specific, an instrument needs to be specific for culture, language and population. When selecting instruments for assessing quality of life, not only is it advantageous to be disease-specific, but also to recognize that the available instruments differ considerably in their scope. Thus the

Table 1 The Karnofsky Index[1]

100%	Normal, no complaints, no evidence of disease
90%	Minor signs
80%	Normal activity with some effort, some signs
70%	Cares for self but unable to carry on normal activity or do normal work
60%	Requires occasional assistance, but is able to care for most of his needs
50%	Requires considerable assistance and frequent medical care
40%	Disabled, requires special care and assistance
30%	Severely disabled, hospitalization is indicated although death is not imminent
20%	Very sick, hospitalization necessary
10%	Moribund, fatal processes progressing rapidly
0%	Dead

McMaster Health Index Questionnaire[7] (MHIQ) assesses emotional parameters as well as social and physical features. In contrast the Hospital Anxiety and Depression (HAD) Scale[8], which was developed for use in physically ill patients, as its name implies, is limited to measuring anxiety and depression. Although measurement of such parameters might well be included in a trial of, for example, advanced breast cancer, it would be insufficient to assess all aspects of the quality of life of such patients.

The Rotterdam Symptom Checklist[9] (which was developed for cancer patients) assesses both physical symptoms such as nausea and pain, and in addition covers sensations likely to be engendered as side-effects of medications, as well as rating psychological adjustment. The Spitzer Quality of Life Index for Cancer Patients[10] is commendably brief, being concise enough to be as acceptable as possible to both clinician and patient by either of whom it can be completed in less than 1 min. It is discriminating and reliable but its brevity results in its omitting several symptoms which are likely to be important in clinical trials, although it embraces occupation, daily living, perception of health, support from family and outlook on life[11]. In contrast, the Nottingham Health Profile[12] is inconveniently, and to many, unacceptably lengthy. It is not specific for malignant disease, indeed it is applicable to healthy as well as sick people, and hence has a role in population surveys. Because it provides a profile of scores it is more sensitive than single figure indices, but having two parts, enquiring about 45 items, repeated administration, as in a clinical trial, is likely to be expensive and monotonous.

The conventional measures of outcome of cancer treatment both within and without clinical trials are entities such as size of tumours, the proportion of respondents and duration of survival. These measures are important, and constitute an essential part of the determination and comparison of efficacy of cancer therapy. It is now recognized that the evaluation of such therapy (particularly when this is for advanced incurable cancer) is incomplete unless it attempts to measure the quality of life. A recently devised concept TWIST (Time Without Symptoms of disease and Toxic effects of Treatment[13]) integrates the chronological with the qualitative measures of outcome. For example, a premenopausal woman treated for locoregional breast cancer by tumourectomy, with axillary clearance (which took 3 weeks), conservation radiotherapy (taking 5 weeks) and a course of six 3 weekly intravenous injections of combination chemotherapy (lasting 18 weeks) commences her TWIST 6 months from date of commencing treatment. Her TWIST may last days, months or years until symptoms caused by relapse, say pain from a bone metastasis, mark its cessation. Local radiotherapy results in complete disappearance of bone pain 1 month after it started. TWIST recommences until the next symptoms occur. The TWIST concept has been further developed by its originators[14] into Q-TWIST (Quality-adjusted TWIST). This enables the total time from onset of treatment to contribute to the final figure. However, it attempts to adjust for impairment of quality of life resulting from side-effects and symptoms by applying 'utility coefficients' which effectively weight for these experiences. Figure 1 shows graphically that Q-TWIST = Ut x TOX + TWIST + Ur x REC. In this example Ut of 0.75 for toxicity and Ur of 0.50 for relapses have been devised arbitrarily. However, it may well be possible to devise these so that they can accurately reflect the impairment of quality of life caused by side-effects of drugs and symptoms of relapse, by using instruments such as those described above. One widely used and well validated technique for quantifying subjective experiences is the Visual Linear Analogue Scale[15,16] which is incorporated into a number of the instruments already described e.g. FLIC[6] and Rotterdam[9]. This simple self-administered method has been shown to be both accurate and reliable in patients with cancer[17]. Although widely accepted methods exist

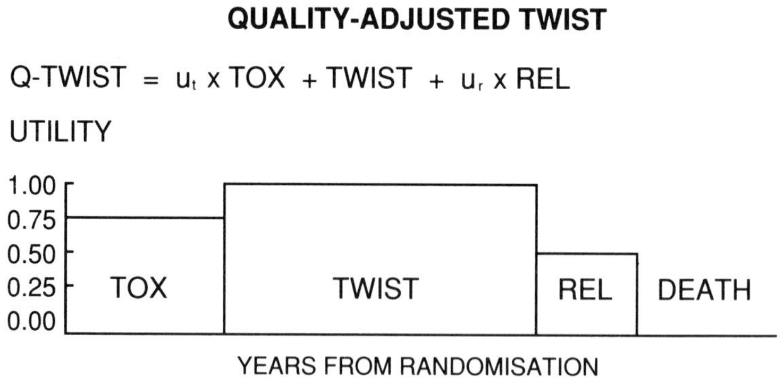

QUALITY-ADJUSTED TWIST

Q-TWIST = u_t x TOX + TWIST + u_r x REL

UTILITY

YEARS FROM RANDOMISATION

Calculation of Q-TWIST: weighted summation of time periods TOX, TWIST and REL. Utility coefficients of ut = 0.75 for TOX and ur = 0.50 for REL are illustrated

Figure 1 Quality-adjusted TWIST (taken from Gelber, R.D., Goldhirsch, A., Simes, R.J., Glaziou, P. and Castiglione, M. (1989)[14], reproduced by kind permission of Springer-Verlag, Berlin)

for analysing scores for linear analogue scales, such scores within a group of patients are not necessarily normally distributed and are usually analysed by logarithmic[16,17] or arc-cosine[17] transformation[18].

That it is necessary to assess the quality of life of patients with breast cancer, (particularly in clinical trials) is indisputable. No perfect instrument has yet been devised to do this. The ideal requirements for such an instrument are that it should be:

(1) Acceptable to patients;
(2) Easy and unambiguous to understand;
(3) Self-administrable and postable;
(4) Sensitive to a wide range of health states;
(5) Capable of repeated administration; and,
(6) Reliably reproducible and statistically evaluable.

"Life alone is not enough –
For there is a kind of slow and weary life
Which is worse than death"

Chinua Achebe in "Arrow of God", 1964
(London: Pan Books Ltd)

REFERENCES

1. Karnofsky, D.A. *et al.* (1948). The use of nitrogen mustards in the palliative treatment of carcinoma. *Cancer*, **1**, 634–56
2. Maddox, G. and Douglas, E.B. (1975). Aging and individual differences: a longitudinal analysis of social, psychological and physiological indicators. *J. Gerontol.*, **29**, 555–63
3. Hunt, S.M., McKenna, S.P., McEwan, J. *et al.* (1981). The Nottingham Health Profile: subjective health status and medical consultations. *Soc. Sci. Med.*, **15A**, 221–9
4. Bergner, M., Bobbit, R.A., Carter, W.B. *et al.* (1981). The Sickness Impact Profile: Development and final revision of a health status measure. *Med. Care*, **19**, 787–805
5. Meenan, R.F. (1982). The AIMS approach to health status measurement: conceptual background and measurement properties. *J. Rheumatol.*, **9**, 785–8

6. Schipper, H. and Levitt, M. (1986). Quality of life in cancer trials: What is it? Why measure it? In Ventrafridda, V., van Dan, F.S.A.M., Yancik, R. *et al.* (eds.) *Assessment of Quality of Life and Cancer Treatment*, pp. 19–29. (Amsterdam: Elsevier Science Publishers)

7. Chambers, L.W. (1982). *The McMaster Health Index Questionnaire (MHIQ): Methodologic Documentation and Report of the Second Generation of Investigations. Department of Clinical Epidemiology and Biostatistics.* (Hamilton: McMaster University)

8. Zigmond, A. and Snaith, P. (1983). The Hospital Anxiety and Depression Questionnaire. *Acta Scand. Psychiatr.*, **67**, 361–8

9. De Haes, J.C.J.M., Van Ostrom, M.A. and Welvaart, K. (1986). The effect of medical and conserving surgery on the quality of life of early breast cancer patients. *Eur. J. Surg. Oncol.*, **12**, 337–42

10. Spitzer, W.O., Dobson, A.J., Hall, J. *et al.* (1981). Measuring the quality of life of cancer patients. *J. Chronic Dis.*, **34**, 595–7

11. Selby, P. (1987). Measuring the quality of life of patients with cancer. In Walker, S.R. and Rossie, R.M. (eds.) *Quality of Life: Assessment and Application*, pp. 181–203. (Lancaster: MTP Press)

12. Hunt, S.M., McEwan, J. and McKenna, S.P. (1985). Measuring health status: a new tool for clinicians and epidemiologists. *J. R. Coll. Gen. Pract.*, **35**, 185–8

13. Gelber, R.D., Goldhirsch, A., Castiglione, M., Price, K., Isley, M. and Coates, A. for the Ludwig Breast Cancer Study Group (1987). Time without symptoms and toxicity: A quality of life orientated endpoint to evaluate adjuvant therapy. In Salmon, S.E. (ed.) *Adjuvant Therapy of Cancer V.*, pp. 455–65 (Orlando: Grune & Stratton)

14. Gelber, R.D., Goldhirsch, A., Simes, R.J., Glasziou, P. and Castiglione, M. (1989). Integration of quality of life issues into clinical trials of breast cancer. In Cavalli, F. (ed.) *Endocrine Therapy of Breast Cancer III*, pp. 27–35. (Berlin: Springer Verlag)

15. Aitken, R.C.B. (1969). Measurement of feeling using visual analogue scales. *Proc. R. Soc. Med.*, **62**, 989–93

16. Bond, A. and Lader, M. (1974). The use of analogue scales in rating subjective feelings. *Br. J. Med. Psychol.*, **47**, 211–18

17. Priestman, T.J. and Baum, M. (1976). Evaluation of quality of life in patients receiving treatment for advanced breast cancer. *Lancet*, **i**, 899–901

18. Selby, P.J. (1985). Measurement of quality of life after cancer treatment. *Br. J. Hosp. Med.*, **33**, 267–71

11

New directions in research on adjuvant therapy in early breast cancer

J.G.M. Klijn and J.A. Foekens

New directions in research regarding adjuvant treatment of patients with early breast cancer concern: (a) (potential) new treatment modalities and (b) better selection of high- and low-risk patients.

(POTENTIAL) NEW TREATMENT MODALITIES

Treatment modalities of potential interest in early breast cancer are summarized in Table 1.

Long-term endocrine therapy is of special interest with respect to adjuvant therapy with tamoxifen in postmenopausal women. There are trials ongoing, comparing the efficacy of long-term treatment (3 to more than 5 years) with that of short-term treatment (1–2 years)[1]. At present too few trials with sufficient follow-up are available to draw any definite conclusions.

New endocrine agents of interest to be used for systemic adjuvant therapy are luteinizing hormone releasing hormone (LHRH) analogues and new antioestrogens. In view of the beneficial long-term effects of surgical castration in premenopausal women, with about 15% difference with the control group after 15 years of follow-up, medical castration by LHRH analogues is currently applied in adjuvant therapy for premenopausal early breast cancer. However, it is at present unknown what the optimal duration of therapy will be. Realistically, better results

Table 1 Treatment modalities of (potential) interest in early breast cancer

Long-term endocrine therapy

New drugs
  New antioestrogens
  LHRH analogues
  Retinoids inducing cell differentiation
  (a) Agents increasing therapeutic effects and/or decreasing toxicity of known cytotoxic drugs (*N*-acyl-dehydroalanines for doxorubicine, leucovorin for 5-fluorouracil)
  (b) Agents that reverse multidrug-resistance (MDR) i.e. verapamil, cyclosporine

New drug regimens
  Preference for anthracycline containing regimens (FAC versus CMF, etc.)
  Sequential chemotherapy
  Sequential chemo-, endocrine therapy
  Sequential chemo-, radiotherapy
  High-dose chemo-, radiotherapy followed by bone marrow rescue in high-risk patients
  Stimulation of tumour cell growth prior to chemotherapy: estradiol recruitment studies
  Drugs interfering with bone (marrow)–tumour cell interaction: APD
  Monoclonal antibodies against membrane antigens or growth factor receptors (anti-EGF-receptors) in micrometastases
  (a) Radiolabeled hormones or growth factors
  (b) Cytostatic drugs linked to growth factors

than those with surgical castration can not be expected. When the duration of treatment is too short worse effects may be experienced compared to those of surgical castration. New antioestrogens might be more effective than tamoxifen and might overcome the occurrence of resistance to tamoxifen[2,3]. A third group of interesting agents are retinoids aiming at induction of cell differentiation and prevention of dedifferentiation of tumour cells to a more malignant status[4]. Retinoids are currently being used in a trial in Milan aiming at prevention of second or contralateral breast cancers[5]. The occurrence of side-effects, especially dry skin and dry mucous membranes during long-term treatment, is a practical problem with this treatment modality.

Agents increasing therapeutic effects and/or decreasing toxicity of known cytotoxic drugs are also of potential interest. The availability of haematological growth factors offers the possibility of using higher doses of chemotherapy. Agents such as verapamil, cyclosporine or buthionine sulfoximine might reverse multidrug resistance (MDR)[6,7]. However, MDR-gene amplification or overexpression of P-glycoprotein has been detected in only a very low percentage of breast cancers[8]. Interestingly, the new antioestrogen toremifene and its metabolites can potentiate doxorubicin activity in MDR breast tumour cells[9]. Also tamoxifen can have a synergistic interaction with doxorubicin[10]. In addition, *N*-acyl-dehydroalanines[11] and leucovorin[12] can also be applied for increasing therapeutic efficacy or decreasing toxicity induced by doxorubicin and 5-fluorouracil respectively.

Testing of new regimens with known drugs is also important. The clinical trial overview[1] indicates cyclophosphamide + methotrexate + 5-fluorouracil (CMF) as the best drug combination, but CMF was mainly compared with single agents or drug combinations without anthracyclines. An overview of Jones[13] on the clinical efficacy of anthracycline-containing regimens demonstrated that for instance 5-fluorouracil + adriamycin + cyclophosphamide (FAC) treatment is superior to CMF. However, well conducted randomized comparative studies (FAC versus CMF) are still needed[14]. Recently sequential administration of different cytostatic agents has been applied and is still under investigation. In view of several observations[10,15,16] that growth inhibitory endocrine therapy can partly abolish the antitumour effect of some cytostatic drugs (melphalan, fluorouracil), by interaction with cellular uptake of cytostatic drugs or with cell kinetics (arrest in G_0G_1 phase of the cell cycle), application of sequential chemoendocrine therapy seems attractive. It was striking to note in the clinical trial overview[1] that tamoxifen reduced the efficacy of chemotherapy in premenopausal early breast cancer (−9% reduction in annual odds of death), while single treatment with tamoxifen reduced the death rate by 21% compared with no adjuvant therapy. Therefore, more trials with tamoxifen, to be started after the last course of adjuvant chemotherapy, are needed. Of potential interest is also the application of high-dose chemotherapy and radiotherapy followed by bone marrow transplantation in high-risk patients[17]. But the relatively high chance of treatment-related deaths and the high costs are discouraging factors.

During the (early) luteal phase compared to the follicular phase of the menstrual cycle, a higher percentage of normal endometrial and breast cells[18] is in the S-phase of the cell cycle. Also breast tumour cells can be stimulated by oestrogens to go from the G_0- to the S-phase of the cell cycle, making them more vulnerable to cytotoxic drugs[19]. Therefore, the relatively good beneficial effects of adjuvant chemotherapy in premenopausal breast cancer patients compared to postmenopausal patients cannot only be explained by the castration effect of chemotherapy, but at least in part by a higher percentage of tumour cell kill during the first cycles of chemotherapy when this chemotherapy was by chance administered during the second half of the menstrual cycle. In addition, later on when cytotoxic-induced amenorrhoea occurs the endocrine effect of medical castration may contribute to the clinical benefit by preventing outgrowth of surviving tumour cells. In cultures of human breast cancer cells (MCF-7) we have found that short-term stimulation with oestradiol and/or insulin can increase the percentage of cells in S-phase from 15 to 60% after 24 h without an increase in absolute cell number[19,20]. Under certain circumstances consecutive administration of doxorubicin after oestrogen recruitment of tumour cells can indeed result in increased cell kill[19]. Also other groups made the same observation with other cytotoxic agents using oestrogens, progestins or growth factors as growth stimulatory agents[10,21–25]. Most clinical studies in advanced disease show a high incidence of complete remissions (about 40%)[25], but the optimal combination of growth stimulatory hormones or factors and cytotoxic drug regimens as well as the optimal duration of treatment are as yet unknown. In the Netherlands a trial (KWF-CKVO 85–09) investigating the principle of oestrogen recruitment of tumour cells before adjuvant chemotherapy is ongoing with at present a median follow-up of 2 years.

Recently it was found that diphosphonates such as (3-amino-1-hydroxypropylidene)-1,1-biphosphonate (APD) decrease osteoclastic activity and delay the occurrence of bone metastases in patients with advanced disease[26]. Therefore, application of diphosphonates in the adjuvant treatment of patients with early breast cancer aiming to prevent the occurrence of bone metastases might be attractive. Whether the incidence of visceral metastasis will increase during such treatment has to be awaited.

Tumour cells have been detected in approximately 20–30% of bone marrow aspirates in patients with early breast cancer[27]. Application of monoclonal antibodies against membrane antigens or growth factor receptors (for instance, anti–epidermal growth factor (EGF) receptors) might be of value for destroying micrometastases or circulating tumour cells. According to the same principle radiolabelled hormones or radiolabelled growth factors or growth factors linked to cytotoxic drugs might be used to detect and to kill tumour cells.

SELECTION OF HIGH- AND LOW-RISK PATIENTS

In the current discussion on application of systemic adjuvant therapy in primary breast cancer identification of high-risk and low-risk patients is a major issue[28]. Several classical[29–32] (tumour size, lymph node status, histopathology, steroid receptor status) and second-generation (proliferation rate, DNA ploidy, oncogenes, growth factor receptors, and some glycoproteins) prognostic factors[29,33–39] are used for making therapeutic decisions (Tables 2 and 3). Because at present no single prognosticator is sufficiently powerful to be used for treatment decisions, some investigators propose to treat every patient with node-negative breast cancer. Some modern factors, such as ploidy and S-phase fraction[29,33] are also difficult to measure, certainly in routine laboratories. However, if all patients with primary cancer were to be treated, many would be treated unnecessarily for only a small potential benefit. This leads to the medical ethical question of what percentage of patients with significant profit of adjuvant therapy is needed to justify overtreatment in the great majority of the patients. Therefore, we need further refinement in our ability to identify high- and low-risk patients.

Table 2 Classical prognostic factors in primary breast cancer

TNM status − tumour size
　　　　　　　　　− lymph node status
　　　　　　　　　− distant metastases

Age, menopausal status
Histopathology − mitotic grade
　　　　　　　　　　− nuclear grade
　　　　　　　　　　− histologic grade

Steroid receptor status (oestrogen and progesterone receptors)

Table 3 New prognostic factors in primary breast cancer

Proliferative index – LI		1985
– % S-phase		1988
DNA ploidy		1987
Oncogenes – amplification		1987
– expression		
Suppressor genes (Rb gene)		1989
Growth factor receptors – EGF-R		1987
– (IGF-1-R)		1988/1989
– SMS-R		1989
Enzymes – cathepsin D (lysosomal)		1988/1989
– aromatase		1989
Oestrogen-inducible heat shock protein hsp 27		1989
Oestrogen-regulated pS2 protein		1989

We have investigated the prognostic and clinical value of the tumour content of receptors for EGF, insulin-like growth factor 1 (IGF-1), somatostatin and the oestrogen-regulated pS2 protein. In our experience IGF-1 receptors showed no prognostic value at all, while tumour EGF receptor levels had only a moderate clinical value[38]. Patients with intermediate EGF receptor contents in their tumours showed the best prognosis, especially in patients with node-positive or oestrogen receptor (ER)-positive tumours. These results are partly conflicting with those of Sainsbury *et al.*[39]. The somatostatin receptor, however, appeared to be of greater clinical value. Recently we found that patients with somatostatin receptor-positive tumours (15% of the samples measured by J.C. Reubi, Bern, Switzerland) had a clearly better relapse-free survival than patients with somatostatin receptor-negative tumours (30% difference after 5 years of follow-up)[38]. But most interesting are our results of a very recent study on pS2 protein performed in cooperation with, among others, the group of P. Chambon (Strasbourg, France). pS2 negativity was associated with a worse prognosis in patients with ER-positive tumours, and in patients with both node-negative as well as node-positive disease. In node-negative breast cancer patients the ER status normally reveals only an

8–10% difference between ER-positive and ER-negative groups in both disease-free and overall survival[29,30]. In this node-negative patient group, other known prognosticators (nuclear grade, tumour size, ploidy, S-phase function and labelling index) showed a difference in disease-free survival after 5 years of follow-up between high- and low-risk patients, varying between 13 and 20%. *Her-2/Neu* oncogene amplification or expression did not even have clinical value in node-negative patients[29]. Based on our series pS2 protein appeared a stronger prognosticator with a difference of 31% between pS2-positive and -negative patients in node-negative patients. In node-positive patients the difference was even 54% for overall survival between high- and low-risk patients after 5 years of follow-up[40].

REFERENCES

1. Early Breast Cancer Trialists' Collaborative Group (1988). Effects of adjuvant tamoxifen and of cytotoxic therapy on mortality in early breast cancer. *N. Engl. J. Med.*, **319**, 1681–92

2. Gottardis, M.M., Jiang, S.-Y., Jeng, M.-H. and Jordan, V.C. (1989). Inhibition of tamoxifen-stimulated growth of an MCF-7 tumor variant in athymic mice by novel steroidal antiestrogens. *Cancer Res.*, **49**, 4090–3

3. Pyrhönen, S., Valavaara, R. and Hajba, A. (1989). High dose toremifene in advanced breast cancer resistant to or relapsed with tamoxifen treatment. *Book of Abstracts 5th European Conference on Clinical Oncology*, abstr. P-0966

4. Costa, A., Malone, W., Perloff, M., Buranelli, F., Campa, T., Dossena, G., Magni, A., Pizzichetta, M., Andreoli, C., del Vecchio, M., Formelli, F. and Barbieri, A. (1989). Tolerability of the synthetic retinoid fenretinide (HPR). *Eur. J. Cancer Clin. Oncol.*, **25**, 805–8

5. Costa, A., Veronesi, U., De Palo, G., Salvadori, B., Coopmans de Yoldi, G., Marubini, E., Formelli, F., Del Vecchio, M. and Rotmensz, N. (1989). Chemoprevention of contralateral breast cancer with fenretinide. *Book of Abstracts 5th European Conference on Clinical Oncology*, abstr. 8-0873

6. Gottesman, M.M. and Pastan, I. (1989). Clinical trials of agents that reverse multidrug-resistance. *J. Clin. Oncol.*, **7**, 409–11

7. Dusre, L., Mimnaugh, E.G., Myers, C.E. and Sinha, B.K. (1989). Potentiation of doxorubicin cytotoxicity by buthionine sulfoximine in multidrug-resistant human breast tumor cells. *Cancer Res.*, **49**, 511–15

8. Merkel, D.E., Fugua, S.A.W., Tandon, A.K., Hill, S.M., Buzdar, A.V. and McGuire, W.L. (1989). Electrophoretic analysis of 248 clinical breast cancer specimens for P-glycoprotein overexpression of gene amplification.

J. Clin. Oncol., **7**, 1129–36

9. DeGregorio, M.W., Ford, J.M., Benz, C.C. and Wiebe, V.J. (1989). Toremifene: pharmacologic and pharmacokinetic basis of reversing multidrug resistance. *J. Clin. Oncol.*, **7**, 1359–64

10. Osborne, C.K., Kitten, L. and Arteaga, C.L. (1989). Antagonism of chemotherapy-induced cytotoxicity for human breast cancer cells by antiestrogens. *J. Clin. Oncol.*, **7**, 710–17

11. Buc-Calderon, P., Praet, M., Ruysschaert, J.M. and Roberfroid, M. (1989). Increasing therapeutic effect and reducing toxicity of doxorubicin by N-acyl dehydroalanines. *Eur. J. Cancer Clin. Oncol.*, **25**, 679–85

12. Swain, S.M., Lippman, M.E., Egan, E.F., Drake, J.C., Steinberg, S.M. and Allegra, C.J. (1989). Fluorouracil and high-dose leucovorin in previously treated patients with metastatic breast cancer. *J. Clin. Oncol.*, **7**, 890–9

13. Jones, S.E., Moon, T.E., Bonadonna, G., Valagussa, P., Rivkin, S., Buzdar, A., Montague, E. and Powles, T. (1987). Comparison of different trials of adjuvant chemotherapy in stage II breast cancer using a natural history data base. *Am. J. Clin. Oncol.*, **10**, 387–95

14. Carbone, P.P. (1989). Doxorubicin as adjuvant therapy for breast cancer: answers or more questions? *J. Clin. Oncol.*, **7**, 554–6

15. Fisher, B., Redmond, C., Brown, A., Fisher, E.R., Wolmark, N., Bowman, D., Plotkin, D., Wolter, J., Bornstein, R., Legault-Poisson, S., Saffer, E.A. and other NSABP Investigators (1986). Adjuvant chemotherapy with and without tamoxifen in the treatment of primary breast cancer: 5-year results form the National Surgical Adjuvant Breast and Bowel Project trial. *J. Clin. Oncol.*, **4**, 459–71

16. Lippman, M.E. (1989). Can oncologists add? *J. Clin. Oncol.*, **7**, 698–9

17. Frei, E., Antman, K., Teicher, B., Edder, P. and Schnipper, L. (1989). Bone marrow autotransplantation for solid tumours – prospects. *J. Clin. Oncol.*, **7**, 515–26

18. Potten, C.S., Watson, R.J., Williams, G.T., Tickle, S., Roberts, S.A., Harris, M. and Howell, A. (1988). The effect of age and menstrual cycle upon proliferative activity of the normal human breast. *Br. J. Cancer*, **58**, 163–70

19. Bontenbal, M., Sonneveld, P., Foekens, J.A. and Klijn, J.G.M. (1988). Oestradiol enhances doxorubicin uptake and cytotoxicity in human breast cancer cells (MCF-7). *Eur. J. Cancer Clin. Oncol.*, **24**, 1409–14

20. Bontenbal, M., Sieuwerts, A.M., Klijn, J.G.M., Peters, H.A., Krijnen, H.L.J.M., Sonneveld, P. and Foekens, J.A. (1990). Effect of hormonal manipulation and doxorubicin administration on cell cycle kinetics of human breast cancer cells. *Br. J. Cancer*, **60**, 688–92

21. Weichselbaum, R.R., Hellman, S., Piro, A.J., Nove, J.J. and Little, J.B.

(1978). Proliferation kinetics of a human breast cancer cell line *in vitro* following treatment with 17-ß-estradiol and 1-ß-D-arabinofuranosyl-cytosine. *Cancer Res.*, **38**, 2339–42

22. Clarke, R., van der Berg, H.W., Kennedy, D.J. and Murphy, R.F. (1985). Oestrogen receptor status and the response of human breast cancer cell lines to a combination of methotrexate and 17-ß-oestradiol. *Br. J. Cancer*, **51**, 365–9

23. Hug, V., Johnston, D., Finders, M. and Hortobagyi, G. (1986). Use of growth stimulatory hormones to improve the *in vitro* therapeutic index of doxorubicin for human breast tumors. *Cancer Res.*, **46**, 147–52

24. Shaikh, N.A., Owen, A.M, Ghilchik, M.W. and Braunsberg, H. (1989). Actions of medroxyprogesterone acetate on the efficacy of cytotoxic drugs: studies with human breast cancer cells in culture. *Int. J. Cancer*, **43**, 458–63

25. Paridaens, R.J., Kiss, R., de Launoit, Y., Atassi, G., Klijn, J.G.M., Clarysse, A., Rotmentz, N. and Sylvester, R.J. (1987). Chemotherapy with estrogenic recruitment in breast cancer. In Klijn, J.G.M., Paridaens, R. and Foekens, J.A. (eds.) *Hormonal Manipulation of Cancer: Peptides, Growth Factors, and New (Anti) Steroidal Agents. EORTC Monograph Series*, vol.18, pp. 477–86. (New York: Raven Press)

26. Van Holten-Verzantvoort, A.T., Bijvoet, O.L.M., Cleton, F.J., Hermans, J., Kroon, H.M. and Harinck, H.I.J. (1987). Reduced morbidity from skeletal metastases in breast cancer patients during long-term biposphonate (APD) treatment. *Lancet*, **ii**, 983–5

27. Mansi, J.L., Berger, U., McDonnell, T., Pope, A., Rayter, Z., Gazet, J.C. and Coombes, R.C. (1989). The fate of bone marrow micrometastases in patients with primary breast cancer. *J. Clin. Oncol.*, **7**, 445–9

28. McGuire, W.L. (1989). Adjuvant treatment of node-negative breast cancer. *N. Engl. J. Med.*, **320**, 525–7

29. McGuire, W.L. (1989). Prognostic factors for recurrence and survival. In *Educational Booklet American Society of Clinical Oncology*, 25th Annual Meeting, pp. 89–92

30. Fisher, B., Redmond, C., Fisher, E.R., Caplan, R. and Other Contributing National Surgical Adjuvant Breast and Bowel Project Investigators (1988). Relative worth of estrogen or progesterone receptor and pathologic characteristics of differentiation as indicators of prognosis in node negative breast cancer patients: findings from National Surgical Adjuvant Breast and Bowel Project Protocol B-06. *J. Clin. Oncol.*, **6**, 1076–87

31. Alexieva-Figusch, J., van Putten, W.L.J., Blankenstein, M.A., Blonk-van der Wijst, J. and Klijn, J.G.M. (1988). The prognostic value and relationships of patient characteristics, estrogen and progestin receptors, and

site of relapse in primary breast cancer. *Cancer*, **61**, 758–68

32. Foekens, J.A., Portengen, H., van Putten, W.L.J., Peters, H.A., Krijnen, H.L.J.M., Alexieva-Figusch, J. and Klijn, J.G.M. (1989). Prognostic value of estrogen and progesterone receptors measured by enzyme immunoassays in human breast tumor cytosols. *Cancer Res.*, **49**, 5823–8

33. Clark, G.M., Dressler, L.G., Owens, M.A., Pounds, G., Oldaker, T. and McGuire, W.L. (1989). Prediction of relapse or survival in patients with node-negative breast cancer by DNA flow cytometry. *N. Engl. J. Med.*, **320**, 627–33

34. Silvestrini, R., Daidone, M.G., Valagussa, P., Di Fronzo, G., Mezzanotte, G. and Bonadonna, G. (1989). Cell kinetics as a prognostic indicator in node-negative breast cancer. *Eur. J. Cancer Clin. Oncol.*, **25**, 1165–71

35. Rochefort, H., Augereau, P., Capony, F., Garcia, M., Cavailles, V., Freiss, G., Morisset, M. and Vignon, F. (1989). The 52K cathepsin-D of breast cancer: structure, regulation, function and clinical value. In Lippman, M.E. and Dickson, R. (eds.) *Breast Cancer: Cellular and Molecular Biology*, pp. 207–23. (Boston: Kluwer Academic Publishers)

36. Silva, M.C., Rowlands, M.G., Dowsett, M., Gusterson, B., McKinna, J.A., Fryatt, L. and Coombes, R.C. (1989). Intratumoral aromatase as a prognostic factor in human breast carcinoma. *Cancer Res.*, **49**, 2588–92

37. Foekens, J.A., Portengen, H., Janssen, M. and Klijn, J.G.M. (1989). Insulin-like growth factor-1 receptors and insulin-like growth factor-1-like activity in human primary breast cancer. *Cancer*, **63**, 2139–47

38. Foekens, J.A., Portengen, H., van Putten, W.L.J., Trapman, A.M.A.C., Reubi, J-C, Alexieva-Figusch, J. and Klijn, J.G.M. (1989). The prognostic value of receptors for insulin-like growth factor-1, somatostatin, and epidermal growth factor in human breast cancer. *Cancer Res.*, **49**, 7002–9

39. Sainsbury, J.R.C., Farndon, J.R., Needham, G.K., Malcolm, A.J. and Harris, A.L. (1987). Epidermal-growth-factor receptor status as predictor of early recurrence and death from breast cancer. *Lancet*, **i**, 1398–1402

40. Foekens, J.A., Rio, M-C., Seguin, P., van Putten, W.L.J., Fauque, J., Nap, M., Klijn, J.G.M. and Chambon, P. (1990). Prediction of relapse and survival in breast cancer patients by pS_2 protein states. *Cancer Res.*, **50**, 3032–7

12

The potential for a novel pure antioestrogen

A.E. Wakeling

INTRODUCTION

All of the antioestrogens available in the early 1980s, including Nolvadex (tamoxifen), show partial oestrogenic agonist activity whose significance in breast cancer treatment cannot be determined[1]. The potential benefit of complete oestrogen withdrawal in breast cancer patients, a goal which is not achieved by aromatase inhibitors or luteinizing hormone releasing hormone (LHRH) analogues, can be evaluated only by clinical trials with a pure antioestrogen. The elimination of partial agonist activity might also reduce the risks of endocrine toxicity associated with the oestrogenic actions of tamoxifen[2], and hence extend the therapeutic indications for antioestrogen therapy to a range of non–malignant conditions. ICI 164,384 (Figure 1) is one of a series of novel antioestrogens, which has been under active investigation for some years and has all the characteristics of a pure antioestrogen.

CHEMISTRY

In seeking to identify novel antioestrogens devoid of oestrogenic activity, a possible lead was offered by observations that 7α analogues of oestradiol, with long alkyl chains, retained a high affinity for the oestrogen receptor[3].

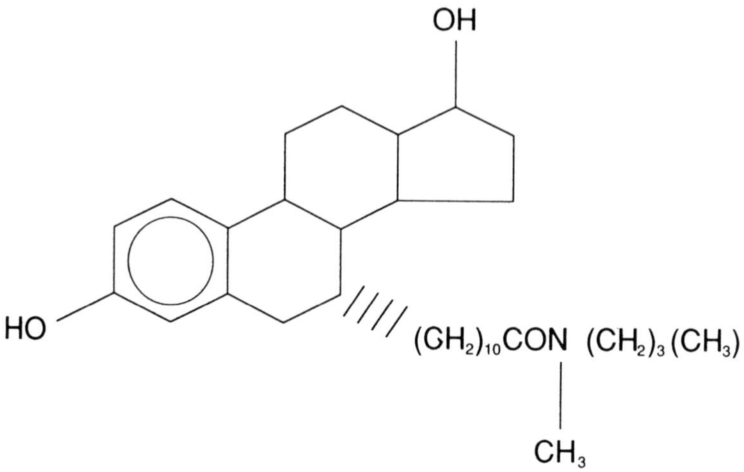

OH

HO

$(CH_2)_{10}CON$ $(CH_2)_3 (CH_3)$

CH$_3$

Figure 1 Structure of ICI 164,384

Synthesis of a series of compounds with a functional group separated from the oestradiol nucleus by a C10 alkyl chain attached at the 7 position of oestradiol produced both classical partial agonists and pure antagonists[4]. The compound of choice for further study was ICI 164,384, a tertiary alkylamide N-n-butyl-11-(3, 17-beta-dihydroxyoestra-1, 3, 5(10)-trien-7α-yl)-N-methylundecanamide (Figure 1).

PHARMACOLOGY

The effect of tamoxifen alone or in combination with oestradiol on the growth of the uterus of immature rats is illustrated in Figure 2a. When given alone, tamoxifen stimulated the growth of the uterus but even at high doses, the maximum stimulatory effect was less than that of oestradiol; this is a characteristic partial agonist (oestrogenic) effect. Correspondingly when animals were treated concurrently with oestradiol and tamoxifen, the uterotrophic action of oestradiol was blocked partially, but not completely. In effect, the expression of the antioestrogenic action of tamoxifen in this model is limited by its inherent oestrogenic activity.

The effect of ICI 164,384 in this assay is shown in Figure 2b. When

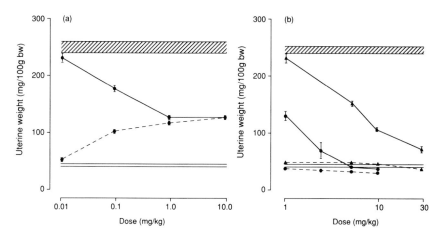

Figure 2 Uterotrophic and antiuterotrophic effects of tamoxifen (a) or ICI 164,384 (b) in immature rats. Animals received three daily doses of vehicle alone (open bar), 0.5 µg oestradiol benzoate alone (hatched bar), or increasing doses of tamoxifen or ICI 164,384 alone (dashed lines) or together with oestradiol benzoate (solid lines) subcutaneously (●) or orally (▲)

administered alone, ICI 164,384 did not stimulate the uterus and, when given concurrently with oestradiol, it blocked the stimulatory activity of the natural hormone completely. Thus, ICI 164,384 is an oestradiol antagonist without intrinsic oestrogenic activity, i.e. it is a pure antioestrogen in this assay. Other studies have shown that unlike tamoxifen, whose effects vary from full agonist, through partial agonist, to pure antagonist in different biological systems, ICI 164,384 is a pure antagonist in every experimental model examined to date[4-6]. ICI 164,384 also blocks the uterotrophic and mammotrophic effects of tamoxifen[5,6].

A most instructive comparison between the effects of ICI 164,384 and tamoxifen was provided by studies in intact rats. Both compounds produced a dose-related reduction of uterine weight, but involution of the uterus in ICI 164,384-treated animals was almost equivalent to that in ovariectomized rats, whereas tamoxifen, even at high doses, achieved a much less effective reduction. An even more dramatic difference was apparent in effects on serum luteinizing hormone (LH) concentration and on the growth of treated animals. Both indices were suppressed significantly by tamoxifen, effects that are due to the central (hypothalamic) oestrogenic activity of tamoxifen. In ICI 164,384-treated

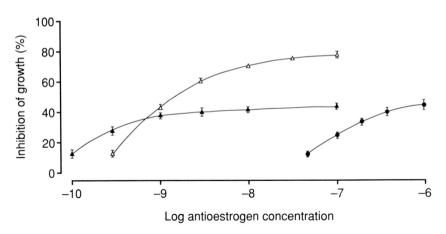

Figure 3 Antioestrogen inhibition of MCF-7 cell growth. Cells were grown for 5 days in Eagle's minimal essential medium containing phenol red, the medium was supplemented with Hanks' salts, non-essential amino acids, L-glutamine, antibiotics, 10 µg/ml insulin and 5% foetal calf serum depleted of endogenous steroids by charcoal treatment. Cells were buffered with bicarbonate and grown in monolayers at 37 °C in an atmosphere of 5% CO_2. Cells were grown in the absence (control) or presence of increasing concentrations of tamoxifen (●), 4-hydroxytamoxifen (▲) or ICI 164,384 (Δ). Growth inhibition was calculated from the ratio of total cell protein in treated and control cultures measured *in situ* on washed cell monolayers using the Lowry method. Each point represents a mean ± SEM for a minimum of six observations

rats no change was seen, compared with intact vehicle-treated controls, indicating the complete absence of any central antioestrogenic or oestrogenic activity, even at doses that blocked peripheral (uterotrophic) action of endogenous oestradiol[4]. A similar peripheral selectivity of action in man would offer considerable therapeutic potential for the treatment of uterine and breast pathology in premenopausal patients, without stimulation of the hypothalamic–pituitary–ovarian axis.

MODE OF ACTION

Classical competitive antagonism between antioestrogens and oestradiol for binding to the high affinity specific oestrogen receptor (ER) *in vitro* is readily demonstrable. Such studies with ICI 164,384 using preparations of ER either from rat[5], human[7] or porcine[8] uterus showed that the affinity

Table 1 Effects of tamoxifen and ICI 164,384 on the population distribution of MCF-7 cells[11]

| | Percentage distribution of cells | | | |
| | Dividing cells | | Non-dividing cells | |
Treatment	G_1	S,G_2,M	G_1	S,G_2,M
Oestradiol 0.1 nM	40	7	51	2
Oestradiol+tamoxifen				
0.1 μM	33	6	58	3
1.0 μM	20	5	72	3
4.0 μM	16	3	77	4
Oestradiol+ICI 164,384				
10 nM	18	4	74	4
0.1 μM	4	2	88	6
1.0 μM	5	3	87	5

of ICI 164,384 for ER is approximately 10-fold greater than that of tamoxifen. Direct studies, using radiolabelled ICI 164,384 and a partially purified preparation of human uterine ER, showed that ICI 164,384 and oestradiol bind to a similar number of sites with comparable affinity[7]. These receptor studies are consistent with the pharmacological properties of ICI 164,384.

Comparative studies of the growth inhibitory action of ICI 164,384 and tamoxifen on MCF-7, ER-positive human breast cancer cells, emphasized the potency advantage of ICI 164,384 over tamoxifen[5]. Of more potential significance was the observation in the former studies that ICI 164,384 was more effective than tamoxifen in reducing the rate of growth of MCF-7 cells. Subsequently, it was shown that this difference did not simply reflect a difference of potency, since 4-hydroxytamoxifen, which has an affinity for ER exceeding that of ICI 164,384[9], was no more effective than tamoxifen. In a standard 5-day growth assay, ICI 164,384 reduced cell number by 80%, compared with a maximum 50% reduction in cultures treated with 4-hydroxytamoxifen or tamoxifen (Figure 3).

Evaluation of cell cycle[10] and population distribution[11] effects showed that both tamoxifen and ICI 164,384 block proliferation of MCF-7 cells in the G1 phase of the cell cycle, but that ICI 164,384 has this effect on a larger proportion of cells (Table 1). Extrapolation of these observations to the therapy of breast cancer would imply that a pure antioestrogen might provide additional benefit in terms of onset, duration or completeness of response in comparison with the action of Nolvadex. This concept remains to be tested clinically.

REFERENCES

1. Nicholson, R.I. (1987). Anti-oestrogens and breast cancer therapy. In Furr, B.J.A. and Wakeling, A.E. (eds.) *Pharmacology and Clinical Uses of Inhibitors of Hormone Secretion and Action*, pp. 60–86. (Eastbourne: Balliere Tindall)
2. Tucker, M.J., Adam, H.K. and Patterson, J.S. (1984). Tamoxifen. In Laurence, D.R., McLean, A.E.M. and Weatherall, M. (eds.) *Safety Testing of New Drugs*, pp. 125–61. (London: Academic Press)
3. Bucourt, R., Vignau, M., Torelli, V. *et al.* (1978). New biospecific adsorbents for the purification of estradiol receptor. *J. Biol. Chem.*, **253**, 8221–8
4. Wakeling, A.E. and Bowler, J. (1988). Biology and mode of action of pure antioestrogens. *J. Steroid Biochem.*, **30**, 141–7
5. Wakeling, A.E. and Bowler, J. (1987). Steroidal pure antioestrogens. *J. Endocrinol.*, **112**, R7–R10
6. Nicholson, R.I., Gotting, K.E., Gee, J. *et al.* (1988). Actions of oestrogens and antioestrogens on rat mammary gland development: relevance to breast cancer prevention. *J. Steroid Biochem.*, **30**, 95–103
7. Weatherill, P.J., Wilson, A.P.M., Nicholson, R.I. *et al.* (1988). Interaction of the antioestrogen ICI 164,384 with the oestrogen receptor. *J. Steroid Biochem.*, **30**, 263–6
8. Wilson, A.P.M., Weatherill, P.J., Nicholson, R.I. *et al.* (1990). A comparative study of the interaction of oestradiol and the steroidal pure antioestrogen, ICI 164,384 with the molybdate-stabilised oestrogen receptor. *J. Steroid Biochem.*, **35**, 421–8
9. Wakeling, A.E. and Bowler, J. (1989). Novel antioestrogens. *Proc. R. Soc. Edinburgh, section b (biological sciences)*, **95**, 247–52
10. Musgrove, E.A., Wakeling, A.E. and Sutherland, R.L. (1989). Points of action of estrogen antagonists and a calmodulin antagonist within the MCF-7 human breast cancer cell cycle. *Cancer Res.*, **49**, 2398–404
11. Wakeling, A.E., Newboult, E. and Peters, S.W. (1989). Effects of antioestrogens on the proliferation of MCF-7 human breast cancer cells. *J. Mol. Endocrinol.*, **2**, 225–34

Discussion II

Professor Mansel

Much as I hate to criticize medical oncologists, I wonder if Mr Lewis would comment on Dr Howell's approach. It was interesting. We were talking about the lumpers and the splitters. It seemed the whole point of the overview was to combine everything to look at it, and then Dr Howell spent the whole of his talk splitting it all up again and looking for the differences. Is that a valid exercise? Secondly, do we really in the 1990s have to be talking about amenorrhoea? Why not just measure the gonadotropins? Why do we not just do these things and swot up the endocrine effects of chemotherapy?

Mr Lewis

I can address the lumping and the splitting. I shall not attempt to address the other issue. I obviously am a lumper by nature rather than a splitter, but that is only from the point of view of drawing conclusions. If I want to do research I split with the best of them. And that is how I regard what Dr Howell was doing. He was splitting in order to generate hypotheses for further work and to try to explain the findings that we have seen, and not draw definitive conclusions. If he was drawing definitive conclusions, then I would have to start to argue with him.

Dr Rose

Before we get too proud of these results, the data have been collected over a period of 7 or 8 years. How many cases of primary breast cancer actually arise in this period? It could be millions. Yet we are very proud that we have collected 30 000 cases. Speaking to Mr Lewis, as a lumper of data, is he not a little worried that there might be a very heavy selection in these 30 000 patients? If for example we look at the British trial, what percentage of the total number of breast cancer cases in Britain are included in the NATO trial? And in the United States the percentage is even smaller. And I could continue in that vein. Do we have any idea of what kind of selection could influence these results? My guess would be that the best patients actually are those who are included in these trials, those patients where one would expect the greatest benefit of any kind of therapy.

Mr Lewis

That is a question that arises in all clinical research that we do. We are always looking for a very small proportion of patients in clinical trials and extrapolating the results to all the patients that we subsequently treat. So one should not regard it as a cancer question. In fact it is probably much worse in other indications in terms of the proportion of patients who get into clinical trials. They are always a selected group and they always will be. The question is whether we can extrapolate the conclusions from selected groups to the population at large. I believe we can, but I base my rationale for this on a way of thinking about clinical research to which perhaps others do not always subscribe. I think of clinical trials as being experiments to test hypotheses, and if the experiment works, then we accept the hypothesis. In other words, I do not think we have to go testing whether gravity works all around the surface of the globe in order to believe in the theory of gravity. We do it once, in one experiment, and that tests our hypothesis about gravity. I feel the same in terms of clinical research. We do an experiment to test our hypothesis. Now that is fine, except for the people who believe, and I know that there are a lot of them, that we should do a cross-sectional study of patients when we do research in order to be able to extrapolate more safely. And the reason that I am less worried than they probably are about that, is that I believe that if we get treatment trends in any particular subgroup of patients they are likely to be in the same direction in other patients. It is the same point

126

as I was making earlier. In other things, I do not think we shall be widely out when we extrapolate to other groups, although we may be out in terms of the exact size of the benefit. But I find it very hard to believe that these results show the effect that they do but that in other patients of other types we shall get an exactly converse result. I may be larger or smaller but I do not think it will be different.

Dr Howell

The 21 years from discovery of Zoladex to getting it into the clinic is absolutely fascinating. It really is a huge investment in time.

Dr Furr

I have a slide of the history of Nolvadex which shows the timescales there, and they are not too dissimilar.

Dr Howell

It is fair to say that Harry Gregory is the man who has missed two Nobel prizes, because he had the structure of epidermal growth factor as well as the structure of LHRH.

Dr Furr

Yes. He has had a very unfortunate life, and he is not particularly well at the moment. He has come incredibly close and he is probably one of the greatest scientists we have had in the company (ICI), and it is nice that you should pay such a tribute to him.

Professor Mansel

Dr Furr described the internalization of receptor, and then we had a nice cartoon and the LHRH agonist waiting for the regeneration receptor. He did not quite explain what the controlling factor is for reproduction of the receptor, because once it is internalized it has presumably to be made and put out again. Can he tell us more about the process?

Dr Furr

I am not sure that a tremendous amount is known about that particular receptor, but for some of the other receptors there are coupling systems. The receptor is made at the same time as the packaging of the LH into granules. There are certainly other receptors in other systems where when the drug is secreted, the hormone is secreted, and the granule fuses with the cell membrane, it redeposits the receptor on the cell surface. But obviously where these things get out of synchronization and a sufficient time is not allowed – there is a finite time; receptor turnover is something like 8–10 hours – to get it back, if it is destroyed completely, and if it gets out of synchronization it cannot be put back in sufficient numbers.

I still think, although I cannot prove it experimentally, that receptor is being deposited on the surface even in cells that are not responding. But we are not developing a big enough quantum of receptors when they get internalized to stimulate a significant response. But it is an area where there is not as much known about the LHRH receptor as there is about the growth hormone receptor, or the LH receptor on the luteal cell where there is a lot more information available.

Dr Howell

The psychiatrists tell us that we must evaluate everything against them. We have evaluated the HADs and we have evaluated the Rotterdam symptom checklist and both of them give 70% specificity and 70% sensitivity. What is the utility of instruments which have that degree of sensitivity and specificity with respect to their use in clinical trials. I am really very worried about the whole process of measurement here. I am suggesting that they are inaccurate.

Mr Preece

That is a problem. I do not know the answer to it, but my gut reaction is that we at least should be trying, and although the tools available to us are inadequate, we at least should be making a gesture to use them and hopefully in practice they would be refined.

Dr Howell

Which of these measures is to be incorporated in Professor Jonat's forthcoming trial?

Professor Jonat

That is a new sheet of paper which we are trying to fill. The problem is always that we have certain subjective effects which can be set, such as vomiting or nausea. But there are other questions, such as 'How do you feel about the treatment?' or 'How do you feel about being ill?', and to get both things on to one sheet of paper is extremely difficult such that the patient can answer them and it will help us in treating the patient.

Dr Howell

The instrument has to be evaluated before it can be incorporated into the trial

Professor Jonat

If I can add something to that. I really doubt that these things do help us. What do they really mean? That we know something more about the treatment procedure. But nonetheless we have to speak with the patient and we have to tell the patient that she can expect such and such from the treatment, or she can expect such and such. We can even set numbers. We can say that one treatment carries the number 9 and another treatment carries the number 7. But nonetheless the patient herself will still agree to what the clinician says.

Dr Howell

Yes. If we tell the patient that what we intend doing is nasty but that it will improve survival, then the patient will accept an enormous amount.

Professor Jonat

So I really doubt that knowing these things is of help to us in the clinical situation.

Dr Howell

You showed our data on the labelling index of the normal breast during the menstrual cycle and that in the second half of the cycle there is an increase in the labelling index. You assumed that the tumour would also show a rise in labelling index due to circulating oestrogens but you have no data to support that.

Dr Klijn

No, but there was a study which showed a clear increase in the labelling index after 3 days of treatment with oestrogens which fell very dramatically following the addition of chemotherapy.

Dr Nicholson

May we know more about the methodology for measuring pS2.

Dr Klijn

It is by radioimmunoassay using two monoclonal antibodies to the protein. These monoclonal antibodies are prepared by Chambon's group and will be available commercially at the beginning of 1990.

Dr Nicholson

Is it possible to do the assay by immunocytochemistry?

Dr Klijn

Yes. There are also studies applying monoclonal antibodies in immunohistochemistry but so far the prognostic value of immunohistochemistry is less than qualitative measurement by radioimmunoassay. At ECCO there was one abstract on the prognostic value of immunohistochemistry with respect to response to endocrine treatment in patients with relapse and they found that in 70 patients investigated that patients with pS2-positive tumours had an objective response in 55% and in an additional 30% of patients stabilization of disease for > 1 year, so that overall there was an 85% effect that lasted for > 1 year in these patients. But for the pS2-negative patients the response rate was about 40%, which was disappointing.

Dr Howell

All of the studies reported in the latter half of the talk are really designed to find factors which we can use to direct our therapies. Particularly we are interested in the node–negative group and trying to select out those who will get a recurrence in the future. As far as the node–negative group is concerned, what are the best factors for selecting out the poor-risk patients?

Dr Klijn

Based on the overview I have shown, I would think the pS2 protein. No doubt.

Dr Howell

In conjunction though with oestrogen and progesterone receptors.

Dr Klijn

Yes. Especially for the oestrogen receptor-positive group that is a very good indicator.

Dr Howell

But with the node-negative patients there were very few who had recurred.

Dr Klijn

Only 4% of the oestrogen receptor-negative patients were positive for the pS2 protein, and according to the results obtained by Harris and his group, for that group maybe the epidermal growth factor receptor is a good discriminant. But in our study it was not so neat as in their study.

Dr Howell

Are epidermal growth factor receptor and pS2 better than grade and vascular invasion?

Dr Klijn

That is dependent on the extension of grading. In general I think it is not the case. I think pS2 is better – it is a positive factor.

Dr Howell

It is more reproducible than grading?

Dr Klijn

Yes. But in Holland there is a group studying a very complicated method for the grading of tumours. It takes at least 3 months to train the technicians and then they can reach quite a reasonable difference between the high-risk and the low-risk patients.

Section III

Postmenopausal patient management of Stage I breast disease

13

Clinical usefulness of prognostic factors

R.W. Blamey

In the United Kingdom there has been a great deal of emphasis on clinical trials. The statisticians try to draw in as many people as possible but the problem with clinical trials is that they give only one answer; to the question 'is radiation necessary after mastectomy?' they give the answer 'no'. Does that mean that every woman does not need to have radiation after mastectomy? It certainly does not and that is the problem of clinical trials.

Breast cancer is a disease in which length of survival can vary enormously depending on the tumour characteristics. In various trials attempts have been made to separate prognosis, e.g. by use of lymph node positivity and negativity. Lymph node involvement shows prognostic separation but is not a very useful factor. A patient who is lymph node-negative will not necessarily survive breast cancer while another who is lymph node-positive will not necessarily die from it.

However, we already have factors which, when used in combination, give a very accurate answer as to whether a patient has metastases or not and whether those metastases are likely to result in death.

Figure 1 illustrates the long-term survival of a series of patients with relatively early breast cancer (stages I and II). Over a 35-year period some patients died very early from the disease; some, typically those with bone metastases, at 10–20 years. The overall survival at 20–25 years was around 20%

Outcome depends on two sets of factors, one 'time-dependent' the other 'intrinsic', i.e. factors of tumour biology. The time-dependent are the size of the tumour and the lymph node involvement. In this series

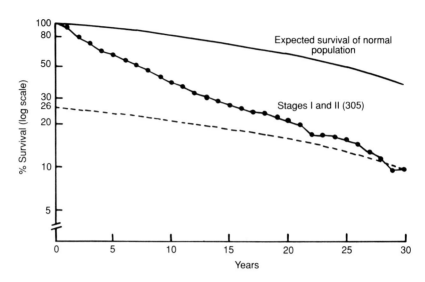

Figure 1 Long-term survival of a series of patients with early breast cancer (stages I and II)

tumour size was measured as the diameter of the fresh specimen. In Nottingham the staging is done by lymph node biopsy at three sites: the low axilla, the high axilla adjacent to the axillary vein and the internal mammary chain through the second interspace. This provides a staging:

(1) Confined to the breast;
(2) Low lymph node involvement; and,
(3) High lymph node involvement.

Many factors are intrinsic but the best at present is certainly (when measured properly) histological differentiation. This is because it probably combines several intrinsic factors; the difficulty is that there are only a few pathologists who can reproducibly grade tumours. Grading in Nottingham has been by Elston's modification of the Bloom and Richardson classification[1]. This incorporates cellular pleomorphism, tubule formation and number of mitoses. Grading is a good prognostic indicator.

Initially nine prognostic factors were assessed for value by multivariate analysis. Such analysis has the value that it eliminates closely related factors. Three factors were found to have independent importance: size, histological grade and lymph node stage.

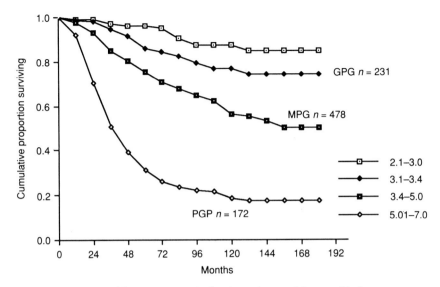

Figure 2   Survival by prognostic index in patients with operable breast cancer

Figure 2 shows the discrimination achieved by the index on survival over a 12-year period. The patient who has a low index has an extremely good chance of long-term survival. The proportion in the Nottingham group is between 20 and 25% of all operable tumours, which equates closely with the percentage long-term survival quoted by Brinkley and Haybittle [2] (Figure 1). The patient with a high index has little chance of being alive after 6 years. Expressing this logarithmically gives the interval probability of dying, another way of expressing the prognosis. Once the prognostic value is assigned there is a constant interval probability of dying as years pass.

The index has been tested in a group of patients prospectively and also by assessing the original group after a longer follow up to determine whether the same factors occur in the multivariate analysis. There were 387 patients in the original group and the index was appplied prospectively in a new group of 320 patients. Comparison of the two groups showed that for each index value the graphs could be superimposed. This confirms that the original prognostic index is accurate. The index can be further improved, e.g. the inclusion of the histological type gives a slightly greater widening of the curve. Other factors can also be investigated such as:

proliferative index measured by flow cytometry, monoclonal antibody staining with an epithelial membrane antibody NCRC 11, epidermal growth factor receptors, oestrogen receptors and lectin binding. All of these show prognostic discrimination but so far when placed in a multivariate analysis have not proved as powerful as histological grade, to which they are related.

Another improvement would be to eliminate the subjectivity of histological grading, possibly by using morphometry in a cell analysis system and combining this with a proliferative index measured in flow cytometry. This appears to give just as good a separation as the pathologists' grading with the advantage that it can be measured objectively by a technician.

It is now possible to make clinical decisions based on the prognostic index. This index separates out a group with a survival probability not significantly different from women without breast cancer who do not need adjuvant therapy. At the other end of the scale is a group with largely undifferentiated tumours who have an extremely poor prognosis; it is reasonable to suggest that chemotherapy is likely to have its best effect as an adjuvant in this group since poorly differentiated tumours are unlikely to respond to hormone therapy. The moderate prognosis group should receive endocrine adjuvant therapy.

Treatment by breast conservation is by no means universally successful and every group is beginning to report local recurrences. In Nottingham slightly different factors are used to separate out an unsuitable group because vascular invasion within the tumour has become an important factor in this. Nevertheless it is the application of a prognostic index to decide which patients are suitable and which are not.

There are various minor points in follow up which should be discussed. A number of hospitals perform bone scans following mastectomy but bone scanning is not as accurate as the prognostic index in indicating whether a patient has occult metastases at the time or not.

The prognostic index can be very useful for giving personal advice. If a young woman asks if she can become pregnant again then we rely heavily on her prognostic factors in telling her what the chances are of her surviving or of her dying and leaving a motherless child.

In the assessment of new treatments it can be useful when it is difficult to carry out randomized trials. The emotion, for example, surrounding the treatment of primary breast cancer in young women means that it is difficult to carry out randomized trials between breast conservation and mastectomy. However, using the prognostic index to stratify the data physicians can get a good idea of what is happening.

These then are the uses of the prognostic index. We must move away from the idea that breast cancer is just a blanket disease that can be treated by one line of treatment. Breast cancers are individual in behaviour.

Once cells have been taken from a cancer it will soon be possible to plot the patient's future; then treatment can be individualized according to the requirements of that particular tumour. This must be the end goal of this research.

REFERENCES

1. Elston, C.W. (1987). Grading of invasive carcinoma of the breast. In Page, D.L. and Anderson, T.J. (eds.) *Diagnostic Histopathology of the Breast*, pp. 300–11. (London: Churchill Livingstone)
2. Brinkley, D. and Haybittle, J.L. (1975). The curability of breast cancer. *Lancet*, **ii**, 95–7

14

Prognostic significance of tumour cell detection in the bone marrow of breast cancer patients at the time of primary therapy

W. Eiermann, N. Harbeck and M. Untch

INTRODUCTION

Breast cancer therapy has seen significant change over the past decades: radical surgery has been replaced more and more by a systemic therapeutic approach. The underlying idea is that breast cancer may be a systemic disease even at a very early stage, although metastatic spread cannot be shown by clinical, radiological or scintigraphical methods at the time of primary therapy. Ultimately one relies on indirect criteria such as tumour size, node status, differential grading, vascular invasion and receptor status to characterize the high-risk patients for systemic disease[1].

These indirect prognostic criteria are the justification for adjuvant chemo- or hormonal therapy.

The results of adjuvant chemotherapy are more disappointing than encouraging after more than 10 years of follow-up to date[2]. According to varying selection criteria, only some patients profit from adjuvant therapy. Therefore the majority of patients undergo considerable side-effects without benefiting from adjuvant therapy. It seems obvious that we need better prognostic criteria to select those patients who are at a high risk of developing metastatic disease.

The skeletal system is a common site for metastases in breast cancer. In two out of three patients it is the site where the initial relapse occurs. By using conventional methods (bone marrow biopsy), only in 3.9% of the cases can distant metastases be detected at the time of primary therapy in patients without metastatic disease[3].

Using immunocytochemical staining methods one can detect tumour cells and clusters in a much higher percentage of bone marrow aspirates. Tumour cell detection increases with the number of sites of aspiration (Table 1).

In this study we evaluated the prognostic significance of bone marrow aspirates for early detection of systemic disease. We aimed to detect tumour cells in the bone marrow of breast cancer patients at the time of primary therapy and to evaluate the presence of such cells in relation to the frequency and site of distant metastases.

Table 1 Detection of tumour cells in the bone marrow: comparison of the results of different research groups

	Patient number	Antibodies	Aspiration sites	Tumour cell detection	
Mansi et al.[8]	307	EMA	8	81	(26.4%)
Eiermann et al.	100	EMA, Cytokeratin, LICR-LON M8	6	33	(33%)
Schlimok et al.[9]	95	CK-2	1	9	(9.5%)
	30	CK-2	2	7	(23%)
Porro et al.[10]	101 (pN0)	MBr-1	1	17	(17%)
	58 (pN1)		(Jamshidi)	8	(14%)
Cote et al.[11]	51	T-16, C-26, AE-1	3	pN0	(27%)
				pN1	(41%)
Manegold et al.[12]	50	Cytokeratin	1	4	(8%)
Ellis et al.[7]	25	Cytokeratin	2	4	(16%)

PATIENTS AND METHODS

From October, 1984 to December, 1988, 105 patients between the ages of 33 and 74 (median 54 years) were studied. In 100 of these patients, distant metastases could not be detected by either clinical, radiological or scintigraphical examination. In the remaining five patients there was clinical suspicion of metastasis at the time of primary therapy. We excluded these five patients from our further statistical evaluations.

Depending on tumour size and clinical node status, all patients underwent either modified radical mastectomy or lumpectomy with axillary node dissection and local irradiation. Independent of the stage of disease, they had bone marrow aspirations performed at six sites (anterior and posterior iliac crest bilaterally, sternum twice) under general anaesthesia immediately after surgery. In the event of lymph node involvement at the time of primary therapy, they received adjuvant systemic therapy afterwards.

From each aspiration site 4–6 ml were taken and placed in heparinized, ice-cold RPMI-1640 (Biochrom, Berlin). With the exception of the first 18 patients, the bone marrow from all sites was pooled. The bone marrow suspension was separated on a Lymphoprep-Isopaque gradient (density 1.077) and further treated according to Böyum's method[4]. This includes further density separation centrifugation, isolation of the interphase layer, further washing, resuspension and again centrifugation. The final suspension was diluted to a concentration of 2×10^7 cells/ml, then smeared on approximately 40 slides, fixed in absolute alcohol and stored at minus 20°C. The slides were later stained according to Dearneley's method[5] except for replacing the polyclonal antibody serum by the following monoclonal antibodies:

(1) Anti-EMA (immunoglobulin (Ig)G2a, clone E-29, Dako, Denmark). This antibody is directed against the epithelial membrane antigen (EMA) of a molecular weight of approximately 265–400 kDa, which was extracted from purified human milk fat globule membranes. It is expressed by almost all epithelial tissues.

(2) LICR-LON M8, which is also a monoclonal antibody against an epitope of the milk fat globule membrane[4].

(3) A cocktail of monoclonal antibodies against Cytokeratin (Moll's catalogue 8, 18, 19 mol. wt.: 39 kDa, 43 kDa, 50 kDa, IgG2a, Becton & Dickinson) and EMA was used starting with patient no. 45.

The slides for the immunocytochemical staining procedure were thawed at room temperature and washed in phosphate-buffered saline. To block the endogenous alkaline phosphatase of the bone marrow cells, 2.28% periodic acid and 20% acetic acid were used. The slides were then incubated with the diluted antibodies in a moist chamber for 60 min at room temperature. After rewashing, the slides were incubated with a rabbit-anti-mouse antibody conjugated to alkaline phosphatase (Dako, Denmark). As a substrate for visualization we used Fast Red TR salt dissolved in Tris buffer pH 8.2 and Naphthol-AS-MX phosphate dissolved in N-N-dimethylformamide, adding 2% Levamisole to block the endogenous alkaline phosphatase again. Afterwards the slides were washed again and counterstained with Mayer's haemalaun and then coverslips were applied. For each patient, a peripheral blood smear was processed after this procedure

To facilitate the screening of the slides we observed them on a monitor connected to an automatic slide table (Prodyscop, Will-Optik, Wetzlar). In addition to immunocytochemical criteria we also used cytological criteria to verify tumour cells and tumour cell clusters. In 19 patients an additional bone marrow biopsy was examined (Professor Bartl, LMU Munich).

As part of their regular follow-up all patients were examined every 3–6 months radiologically (chest X-ray, bone scan) as well as clinically glutamic oxaloacetic transaminase (GOT), glutamic pyruvate transaminase (GPT), γ-glutamyl transpeptidase (γ-GT), carcinoembryonic antigen (CEA) and (CA 15-3).

RESULTS

The multiple bone marrow aspirations under general anaesthesia caused no complications. The aspirates of the first 18 patients were processed separately for each aspiration site. Since there was no significant difference in the distribution of the tumour cells among the sites, the aspirates of the multiple aspiration sites for each patient were subsequently pooled.

The detection of tumour cells was independent of the antibody used, but with the cocktail of anti-Cytokeratin and anti-EMA the staining intensity and detection rate were considerably raised.

Table 2 shows pathological, biochemical and clinical data in relation to the presence of tumour cells in the bone marrow. In 33/100 (33%) patients with metastases-free disease, tumour cells were detected in the bone marrow at the time of primary therapy. In five cases with suspected metastases, we could verify the presence of tumour cells immunocyto-chemically. We were able to detect tumour cells at a limit of one tumour cell in 10^7 bone marrow cells.

There was no significant relation between tumour size, node status, menopausal status and the detection of tumour cells in the bone marrow. Tumour cells were detected in fewer receptor-positive tumours.

Seventeen of the 33 tumour-cell-positive patients (52%) relapsed within a median follow-up period of 24 months (minimum 3, maximum 50 months). Out of the remaining 67 tumour cell-negative patients only seven (10%) relapsed within the same period (Table 3).

Table 2 Relation between the detection of tumour cells in the bone marrow and other prognostic factors (100 patients)

		Tumour cell-positive (n = 33)		Tumour cell-negative (n = 67)	
pT1	(n = 38)	12	(32%)	26	(68%)
pT2	(n = 36)	10	(28%)	26	(72%)
pT3	(n = 4)	1		3	
pT4	(n = 10)	5		5	
pTx	(n = 12)	5		7	
pN0	(n = 33)	12	(36%)	21	(64%)
1–3 lymph nodes	(n = 30)	9	(30%)	21	(70%)
> 3 lymph nodes	(n = 27)	8	(30%)	19	(70%)
pNx	(n = 10)	4		6	
Estrogen receptor:					
positive	(n = 45)	11	(24%)	34	(76%)
negative	(n = 34)	14	(41%)	20	(59%)
not tested	(n = 21)	8		13	
Premenopausal	(n = 41)	12	(29%)	29	(71%)
Postmenopausal	(n = 59)	21	(36%)	38	(64%)
Deceased	(n = 12)	8		4	

Table 3 First location of distant metastases

	Tumour cell-positive (n = 33)	Tumour cell-negative (n = 67)
Bone metastases	11	0
Visceral metastases	1	3
Soft tissue (lymph nodes, skin)	2	3
Mixed	3	1
Total	17 (71%)	7 (29%)

Median follow-up 24 months

In 11 of the 17 tumour cell-positive patients, the first manifestation for distant metastases was in the skeletal system, in eight of 11 in the skeletal system exclusively. Three patients showed combined visceral and skeletal manifestations. The median disease-free time between aspiration and relapse was 7.4 months (minimum 3, maximum 24 months). Of the tumour cell-positive patients, eight are already deceased in comparison to four of the tumour cell-negative patients.

None of the seven tumour cell-negative patients had the skeletal system as a first site of metastases; however, one patient relapsed with visceral as well as bone metastases simultaneously. Three of the remaining six patients in this group had visceral metastases and three had skin metastases of contralateral lymph node metastases.

Table 4 compares conventional histology (bone marrow biopsy) with immunocytochemical staining (bone marrow aspiration). It is remarkable that in only two of 20 patients were tumour cells detected histologically, whereas in 33/100 patients tumour cells were detected immunocyto-chemically.

Table 5 shows this comparison in five patients where metastases were proven by different means. None of the patients with a positive bone marrow biopsy had a negative aspiration. No tumour cells could be found in the immunocytochemically stained peripheral blood smears.

Table 4 Comparison of bone marrow biopsy ($n = 20$) and bone marrow aspiration ($n = 100$) in M0 patients

Stage	Tumour cell-positive	Myelotomy-positive
T1–3 N0 M0 $n = 33$	12 (36%)	1/5
T1–4 N1–2 M0 $n = 67$	21 (31%)	1/15

Table 5 Comparison of myelotomy and bone marrow aspiration in patients with proven metastases ($n = 5$)

Immunocytochemistry	Myelotomy-positive	Myelotomy-negative
Tumour cell-positive	2	3
Tumour cell-negative	0	0

DISCUSSION

The assumption of micrometastases at the time of primary therapy – though with conventional methods (X-ray, bone scan) these could not be detected – is the basis of adjuvant therapy strategies in breast cancer. Whether circulating tumour cells or already existing micrometastases lead to a general spreading of the disease is still under discussion. The detection of micrometastases at the time of primary therapy was limited by the low detection rate by conventional staining techniques in bone marrow aspirates or biopsies. The application of monoclonal antibodies to bone marrows in the search for micrometastases in solid tumour patients clearly enhanced the detection rate in primary breast cancer (see Table 1). Though there are still numerous technical limitations, the principle of this technique is widely accepted.

The technical considerations include the type of antibody used, number of aspiration sites and staining techniques to block endogenous enzyme activity in marrow cells. Particularly if the assay depends on this enzyme, the antibody used is also a critical factor. Dearneley et al.[5] used a polyclonal anti-EMA antibody in their bone marrow evaluation.

Unfortunately, EMA has subsequently been demonstrated to be expressed by non-epithelial cells, including lymphoid cells[6].

Though EMA is also a less sensitive marker of epithelial differentiation than cytokeratins, this antibody seems to be more sensitive in detecting epithelial tumour cells in the bone marrow. Ellis *et al.*[7] however, identified in a small number of patients just two cells in bone marrow specimens that were morphologically clearly plasma cells and that reacted with an anti-cytokeratin antibody. Comparing the detection results published by several groups the detection rates were considerably higher (see Table 1) when a panel of antibodies was used compared with one antibody alone. Another important point is the number of aspiration sites. At least three aspiration sites are necessary (sternum + iliac crest) to enhance the tumour cell detection. The lowest rates of detection were published by those groups who used only one aspiration site. Based on our results and the results of other groups, there may well have been an unknown degree of false positive immunostaining. This, however, would not account for the statistical significance of correlation with clinical outcome. Most published papers show no statistically significant relationship with known prognostic factors, such as lymph node involvement, receptor status and tumour size. However, in most studies the number of patients examined is small. Mansi *et al.*[8] showed a positive relationship between bone marrow involvement and receptor status, lymph node status and tumour size. We are not able to confirm this experience totally. In our data there is a correlation only between oestrogen receptor status and bone marrow involvement. Our follow-up data show bone marrow involvement as a prognostic factor with high significance in predicting bone relapse (see Table 3). In our study, after a median follow-up of 24 months, the risk of bone relapse in patients with bone marrow involvement at primary therapy was significantly higher. According to our data bone relapse was not found in patients who showed no bone marrow involvement at primary therapy. It is now a widely recommended consideration to use adjuvant therapy in all node-negative patients due to favourable data. Node-negative patients who are at high risk for relapse are not yet clearly defined. Bone marrow involvement might characterize those patients which are at high risk for at least bone relapse in a node-negative situation at primary therapy. The optimal role of antibody staging of bone marrows in both low-risk and high-risk breast cancer patients remains still to be determined and merits further studies.

REFERENCES

1. Coombes, R.C., Powles, T.J., Gazet, J.C. *et al.* (1980). Assessment of biochemical tests to screen for metastases in patients with breast cancer. *Lancet*, **i**, 296–8

2. Bonadonna, G. and Valagussa, P. (1985). Adjuvant systemic therapy for resectable breast cancer. *J. Clin. Oncol.*, **3**, 259–75

3. Riddell, B. and Landys, K. (1979). Incidence and histopathology of metastases of mammary carcinoma in biopsies from the posterior iliac crest. *Cancer*, **4**, 1782–8

4. Böyum, A. (1976). Isolation of lymphocytes, granulocytes and macrophages. *Scand. J. Immunol.*, **5** (Suppl.5), 9

5. Dearneley, D.P., Ormerod, M.G., Sloane, J.P. *et al.* (1983). Detection of isolated mammary carcinoma cells in marrow of patients with primary breast cancer. *J. R. Soc. Med.*, **76**, 359–64

6. Untch, M., Harbeck, N. and Eiermann, W. (1988). Micrometastases in bone marrow in patients with breast cancer. *Br. Med. J.*, **296**, 290

7. Ellis, G., Ferguson, M., Yamanaka, E. *et al.* (1989). Monoclonal antibodies for detection of occult carcinoma cells in bone marrow of breast cancer patients. *Cancer*, **63**, 2509–14

8. Mansi, J.L., Berger, U., Easton, D. *et al.* (1987). Micrometastases in bone marrow in patients with primary breast cancer: evaluation as an early predictor of bone metastases. *Br. Med. J.*, **295**, 1093–6

9. Schlimok, G., Funke, I., Holzmann, B. *et al.* (1987). Micrometastatic cancer cells in bone marrow: *in vitro* detection with anti-cytokeratin and *in vivo* labeling with anti-17-1A monoclonal antibodies. *Proc. Natl. Acad. Sci., USA*, **84**, 8672–6

10. Porro, G., Menard, S., Tagliabue, E. *et al.* (1988). Monoclonal antibody detection of carcinoma cells in bone marrow biopsy specimens from breast cancer patients. *Cancer*, **61**, 2407–11

11. Cote, R.J., Hakes, T.B., Bazinet, M. and Old, L.J. (1988). Monoclonal antibodies detect occult breast carcinoma metastases in the bone marrow of patients with early stage disease. *Am. J. Surg. Pathol.*, **12**, 333–40

12. Manegold, C., Krempien, B., Kaufman, M. *et al.* (1988). The value of bone marrow examination for tumor staging in breast cancer. *J. Cancer Res. Clin. Oncol.*, **114**, 425–8

15

The rationale and results of systemic adjuvant therapy in postmenopausal women with stage I breast cancer, including NSABP protocol B-14 (1989)

P.E. Preece

After decades of debate about which type of mastectomy gave the best results in the treatment of breast cancer, it came to be realized that differences in locoregional procedures made marginal if any difference to overall survival, because the vast majority of patients with this disease died from systemic spread[1]. Thus, the rationale for adjuvant systemic therapy emerged, with the key feature being that however or whatever was given, it was commenced at a point close in time to the primary treatment. With Stage II breast cancer having an overall 10-year survival of 40%, it is immediately evident that a modality of treatment which might improve such poor figures should be tried, for in a crude sense, over half the affected patients stand to benefit. It is less easy to see the rationale for systemic adjuvant therapy in Stage I breast cancer with its overall 80% 10-year survival. However, long-term follow-up studies of patients with this disease have shown that it can recrudesce and kill beyond, as well as before, 5 years following initial therapy, these delayed deaths always being attributable to systemic rather than local disease. Bernard Fisher, in his preamble to the preliminary results of NSABP protocols B-13 and B-14, which investigate systemic adjuvant therapy in node-negative operable breast cancer, cites two previous NSABP studies of early disease, in one of which 15% of patients died during the first 5 years of follow-up, and another in which 32% died after 10 years follow-up[2,3].

For the purpose of this paper, the term 'stage I' has been regarded as synonymous with 'node-negative', since the latter term has been used more frequently as a criterion for case selection and stratification in published clinical trials than the term 'stage I'. Information has been taken from 12 major clinical trials of systemic adjuvant therapy which included postmenopausal women with stage I breast cancer (Table 1). Where these trials also recruited premenopausal node-negative women, results for these have been included.

One of the earliest studies was conducted between 1957 and 1963 by Nissen-Meyer[4] who gave the results as a poster at the 1989 meeting of the European Congress of Clinical Oncology held in London. A series of 169 node-negative women was included in this study which compared the addition of radiation menopause to mastectomy with surgery alone. After a mean follow-up interval of 30 years there is a 63% survival in the treated group compared with a 43% survival in the controls. Moreover, the premenopausal node-negative subjects who had a radiation menopause had an incidence of contralateral breast cancer of 2.6% compared with 12.7% in the controls. The same authors, reporting for the Scandinavian Adjuvant Chemotherapy Study Group, evaluated single agent cyclophosphamide given perioperatively[5]. A significantly improved relapse-free and overall survival has persisted for up to 20 years following the therapy. The benefits were observed in both pre- and postmenopausal women, and in node-negative as well as node-positive patients. A further Scandinavian study compared a short course of perioperative combination chemotherapy (cyclophosphamide+methotrexate+5-fluorouracil; CMF) with a 12-month course of the same[6] but excluded node-negative patients from the longer term option. However, comparison of the performance of the node-negative cases with single agent is indistinguishable from that

Table 1 Twelve trials which yield information about systemic adjuvant therapy in node-negative breast cancer

Nissen-Meyer[4]	SCTO[12]
Scandinavian ACSG I[5,6]	Naples (GUN)[13]
Scandinavian ACSG II[7]	Ludwig[14]
Christie[8]	ECOG (Intergroup)[15]
NATO[9,10]	NSABP B-13[2]
CRC[11]	NSABP B-14[3]

of such cases treated with the short multidrug course[7]. Both the short duration (perioperative) regimens, whether single or combination, were much more easily tolerated than the multicycle course.

The 10-year results of the Christie adjuvant tamoxifen trial[8] which included both pre- and postmenopausal patients are particularly interesting for the fact that the most marked trend was in favour of tamoxifen, compared, for premenopausal women in this trial, with radiation menopause. The 10-year survival for the premenopausal tamoxifen-treated women is 93% compared with 82% for those whose ovaries were irradiated. The node–negative postmenopausal women had a similar overall survival at 10 years to controls, but with a consistent trend in favour of tamoxifen, as demonstrated by log rank analyses of first events (death or relapse). In this trial tamoxifen was given for only 1 year. Had it been used for longer, greater benefit may have resulted. The trial of tamoxifen as single adjuvant agent in the management of early breast cancer conducted by the Nolvadex Adjuvant Trial Organization (NATO)[9] included 604 node–negative and 371 node–positive post-menopausal women (and only 128 premenopausal women, none of whom was node–negative). At the 6-year analysis[9] the 300 tamoxifen-treated women had experienced 50 events compared with 73 events in the 305 postmenopausal node–negative controls, a statistically significant difference, which persisted at the 8-year analysis, by which time only 80 events had occurred in the 300 treated with tamoxifen, compared with 107 in the 305 controls[10].

A direct comparison of 6 days of cyclophosphamide with 2 years of tamoxifen has been made by the Cancer Research Campaign Adjuvant Breast Trial Working Party. The preliminary analysis was done when the median follow-up was 40 months[11]. Both cyclophosphamide and tamoxifen resulted in statistically significant observed/expected (O/E) ratio of events for all the treated node–negative patients, both pre- and postmenopausal, compared with untreated controls. This is a substantial study of 2230 women, although of these, 1912 were eligible for this analysis, 60% of whom were node–negative, and 70% of whom were postmenopausal. This study shows no significant advantage of adding cyclophosphamide to tamoxifen. It points to the possibility that adjuvant tamoxifen may protect against contralateral breast cancer.

The first report of the Scottish Trial of adjuvant tamoxifen was published in 1987[12] when the median duration of therapy was 47 months.

One almost unique feature of this trial is that the randomization was between immediate adjuvant tamoxifen for 5 years versus tamoxifen used at first recurrence. For those initially randomized to tamoxifen, secondary randomization has been performed at 5 years between stopping or continuing tamoxifen indefinitely. Of a total of 1323 patients entered, 751 were node-negative, of whom 539 were postmenopausal (and 212 premenopausal). Table 2 shows the percentage of all these (pre- and postmenopausal) surviving at the maximum available follow-up interval at time of publication. The onset of recurrence has been significantly delayed by immediate adjuvant tamoxifen in these node-negative patients (Table 3) (as also in the node-positives). Interestingly, the survival from recurrence in these node-negative patients was less in those who received immediate tamoxifen, namely 17.8 months compared with 24.3 for those given this drug at time of recurrence. This may be explained by the fact that earlier recurrence is a feature of poor prognosis, which is also expressed by oestrogen receptor negativity, i.e. reduced likelihood of being hormone-dependent.

Table 2 Percentage of node-negative patients surviving at maximum available follow-up at time of publication; in Scottish Adjuvant Tamoxifen Trials[12]

	Tamoxifen	*Observed*
Disease-free	74.2	57.0
Survived from randomization	79.3	74.1

Table 3 Numbers and sites of first relapses in node-negative patients by randomized option; in Scottish Adjuvant Tamoxifen Trials[12]

	Tamoxifen	*Observed*
Contralateral	6	11
Locoregional	18	42
Locoregional and systemic	8	12
Systemic	29	39
Total	61	104

A further randomized trial of immediate tamoxifen for 2 years versus no adjuvant therapy, done by the Group of the University of Naples (GUN)[13] included 173 node-negative women who were both pre- and postmenopausal. At a median observation period of 63 months, tamoxifen produced a significant improvement in disease-free survival which did not depend on menopausal status. This study has not been running for a sufficient length of time for a large enough number of events to have occurred to determine if any significant difference in overall survival will be demonstrated.

A number of studies report the effect of systemic adjuvant therapy used specifically for node-negative disease. One such, that of the Ludwig Breast Cancer Study Group[14] studied 1275 node-negative, pre- and postmenopausal breast cancer patients, randomized between no adjuvant therapy and a single course of combination CMF given over 8 days commencing on the second day after mastectomy. The treated women, both pre- and postmenopausal had an advantage, with a mean 4-year disease-free survival of $77 \pm 2\%$ compared with $73 \pm 2\%$ for the controls. Further, the 4-year survival rate showed a trend in favour of the treated subjects (90% cf. 86%). Interestingly the magnitude of the treatment effect was greater in those with low or no oestrogen receptor (i.e. those with most to gain).

The finding of a greater magnitude of treatment effect in a stratum of node-negative patients who were characterized by an unfavourable prognostic determinant has led on to studies which set out to evaluate the effects of systemic adjuvant therapy in 'high-risk' node-negative patients. An ECOG Intergoup Study[15] randomized 536 such node-negative women with oestrogen receptor-negative tumours of any size and oestrogen receptor-positive tumours more than 3 cm in diameter, to six cycles of CMF versus no treatment observation. At a median follow-up of 36 months, the disease-free survival of treated patients was 84% compared with 69% for those patients who were observed only, which is a highly significant difference. Only 10% of treated patients had severe toxicity, and there was one death. An effect on overall survival has not yet been observed.

The NSABP trials B-13[2] and B-14[3] evaluated respectively receptor-negative, node-negative tumours, and receptor-positive, node-negative tumours. In B-13 the comparison was between combination chemotherapy (sequential methotrexate and fluorouracil) and nothing, whereas in B-14 nothing was compared with tamoxifen 10 mg b.d. for 5 years. In B-13, at 4 years, treatment failure was reduced by 24% in premenopausal patients and 50% in postmenopausal patients, and side-effects were tolerable. In B-14 the greatest reduction in treatment failure at 4 years was 44% in the under 50s and 14% in the over 50s. In neither trial B-13 nor B-14 has a significant advantage in overall survival yet been demonstrated, although this may change with the passage of time, since the numbers of subjects from whom data were available for this evaluation represented only a very small proportion of all the eligible and randomized patients. Flushes, menstrual irregularities, phlebitis and vaginal discharge occurred more often in tamoxifen-treated patients; but the numbers were a small proportion of all treated subjects. The major overview of trials of systemic adjuvant tamoxifen and cytotoxic therapy by Peto[16] concluded, for stage I breast cancer, that although there is a reduction in recurrence-free survival when adjuvant therapy is given, so far there is no statistically significant mortality reduction when the analysis is restricted to the node-negative subjects.

Although Fisher *et al.* have used steroid receptors to distinguish high- and low-risk, node-negative breast cancers, they have demonstrated that another prognostic factor, namely nuclear grade, is a better determinant of outcome than the receptors[17]. Others have shown that a combination of tumour size and mean nuclear area gives additional prognostic information[18]. Other readily available prognostic determinants such as serum markers[19] or cytosolic markers[20] may improve the ability to select which node-negative patients might benefit from systemic adjuvant therapy, and may even indicate the duration, intensity and type to achieve optimal effects.

In conclusion, there is incontrovertible evidence that stage I (i.e. nominally good prognosis) breast cancer patients can benefit from systemic adjuvant therapy. Further studies must use the many readily available prognostic factors to determine the high-risk women who may benefit most, and for whom the costs and risks of adjuvant therapy are most worth taking. Finally, these studies must incorporate meticulous measures of the effects, both subjective and objective, both short-term and long-term of the agents used as adjuvant therapy to check that any advantages achieved are not counteracted by accompanying but sometimes obscure disadvantages.

REFERENCES

1. Fisher, B., Bauer, M., Margolese, R. *et al.* (1985). Five year results of a randomized clinical trial comparing total mastectomy and segmental mastectomy with and without radiation in the treatment of breast cancer. *N. Engl. J. Med.*, **312**, 665–73

2. Fisher, B., Redmond, C., Dimitrou, N.V. *et al.* (1989). A randomized clinical trial evaluating sequential methotrexate and fluorouracil in the treatment of patients with node negative breast cancer who have oestrogen receptor negative tumours. *N. Engl. J. Med.*, **320**, 473–8

3. Fisher, B., Costantino, J., Redmond, C. *et al.* (1989). A randomized clinical trial evaluating tamoxifen in the treatment of patients with node negative breast cancer who have oestrogen receptor positive tumours. *N. Engl. J. Med.*, **320**, 479–84

4. Nissen-Meyer, R. (1975). Ovarian suppression and its supplement by additive hormonal treatment. *Inserm*, **55**, 151–8

5. Nissen-Meyer, R., Kjellgren, K., Malmio, K., Mansson, B. and Norin, T. (1978). Surgical adjuvant chemotherapy: results with one short course with cyclophosphamide after mastectomy for breast cancer. *Cancer*, **41**, 2088–98

6. Nissen-Meyer, R., Kjellgren, K. and Mansson, B. (1982). Adjuvant chemotherapy in breast cancer. *Rec. Results Cancer Res.*, **80**, 142–8

7. Nissen-Meyer, R., Host, H., Kjellgren, K., Mansson, B. and Norin, T. (1984). Scandinavian trials with a short post-operative course versus a 12-cycle course (of cyclophosphamide). *Rec. Results Cancer Res.*, **96**, 48–54

8. Ribeiro, G. and Swindell, R. (1988). The Christie Hospital adjuvant tamoxifen trial – status at 10 years. *Br. J. Cancer*, **57**, 601–3

9. Baum, M., Brinkley, D.M., Dossett, J.A. *et al.* (1985). Controlled trial of tamoxifen as single adjuvant agent in management of early breast cancer. Analysis at six years by Nolvadex Adjuvant Trial Organization. *Lancet*, **i**, 836–40

10. Baum, M., Brinkley, D.M., Dossett, J.A. *et al.* (1988). Controlled trial of tamoxifen as a single adjuvant agent in the management of early breast cancer. Analysis at eight years by Nolvadex Adjuvant Trial Organization. *Br. J. Cancer*, **57**, 608–11

11. Abram, W.P., Baum, M., Berstock, D.A. *et al.* (1988). Cyclophosphamide and tamoxifen as adjuvant therapies in the management of breast cancer. Preliminary Analysis by the CRC Adjuvant Breast Trial Working Party. *Br. J. Cancer*, **57**, 604–7

12. Stewart, H.J., White, G.K. *et al.* (1987). Scottish Cancer Trials Office. Adjuvant tamoxifen in the management of operable breast cancer: the Scottish trial. *Lancet*, **ii**, 171–5

13. Bianco, A.R., De Placido, S., Gallo, C. *et al.* (1988). Adjuvant therapy with tamoxifen in operable breast cancer. Lancet, **ii**, 1095–9

14. Ludwig Breast Cancer Study Group (Goldhirsch and Gelber) (1989). Prolonged disease free survival after one course of perioperative adjuvant chemotherapy for node negative breast cancer. *N. Engl. J. Med.*, **320**, 491–6

15. Mansour, E.G., Gray, R., Shatila, A.H. *et al.* (1989). Efficiency of adjuvant chemotherapy to high risk node negative breast cancer. *N. Engl. J. Med.*, **320**, 485–90

16. Peto, R. (1988). Effects of adjuvant tamoxifen and of cytotoxic therapy on mortality in early breast cancer. An overview of 61 randomized trials among 28,896 women. *N. Engl. J. Med.*, **319**, 1681–92

17. Fisher, B., Redmond, C., Fisher, E.R. and Caplan, R. (1988). Relative worth of oestrogen or progesterone receptor and pathologic characteristics of differentiation as indicators of prognosis in node negative breast cancer patients: findings from the NSABP Protocol B-06. *J. Clin. Oncol.*, **6**, 1076–87

18. Maehle, B.O., Skjaerven, R. and Collett, K. (1988). Prognosis in node negative breast cancer patients: the importance of tumour diameter and mean nuclear area. *Eur. J. Surg. Oncol.*, **14**, 21–6

19. Browning, M.C.K., McFarlane, N.P., Horobin, J.M., Preece, P.E. and Wood, R.A.B. (1988). Evaluation of the comparative clinical utility of CA15–3 and MCA in the management of breast carcinoma. *Ann. Clin. Biochem.*, **25** (Suppl. 1), 54–6

20. Tandon, A., Clark, G., Chirgwin, J. and McGuire, W. (1989). Cathepsin D predicts relapse and survival in node–negative breast cancer. *Proc. Am. Assoc. Cancer Res.*, **30**, 352

16

Rationale for treatment of benign breast disease

R. Mansel

Readers may wonder why benign disease should be discussed in a book that has concentrated exclusively on breast cancer. There are various reasons why it might be useful. Many of us, certainly the surgeons and physicians, do see a large number of patients who come to us but who turn out not to have breast cancer, and some of these may require treatment. Secondly, an understanding of what is going on in the benign world and the processes within the breast may well help us to understand what is going on in the malignant breast. For these reasons it might be interesting to look at whether some useful information can be derived from benign disease. There is very little information, despite a number of people concentrating on the problem for many many years. The work described here comes mostly from our centre in Cardiff.

The history of people looking at benign disease goes back an extremely long way. Sir Astley Cooper (noted for Cooper's 'Suspensory Ligaments of the Breast') wrote about this subject many years ago. He commented on breast cysts and also on symptoms within the breast in cases that were not malignant. It should be mentioned that the rationale for treating some cases of benign disease, but not all, is that sometimes symptom relief must be offered to some patients who get severe breast symptoms. Physicians should think in terms of reducing symptoms from the very common cystic disease and, speculatively in terms of reducing proliferative disease which is a risk factor for malignancy.

SYMPTOMS

Many women have no breast pain. Some women have a small amount and would regard it as entirely normal. There are groups of women who have prolonged patterns of pain and these women have menstruation with 3 days of freedom from symptoms, and then for the whole of the rest of the month they have severe breast pain. However, they do not make up a large proportion of the population that attends a breast clinic.

The reasons why one woman has pain when another woman does not have pain are totally unclear, but because of the frequent relationship of pain with the menstrual cycle and ovulation, we all suspect that it has something to do with hormones. However, which hormone and what is wrong, nobody is quite clear about.

Many people have searched for the answer. Mauvais Jarvis has suggested that the problem is a deficient luteal phase leading to a relative hyperoestrogenism. This is a very attractive theory in many ways. It is certainly known that oestrogen is involved in rodent breast problems. Whether it is involved in human breast problems is harder to prove. The data looked quite convincing as there were large differences in luteal function in his control group compared with the disease group. Unfortunately nobody has managed to validate this work. In Cardiff salivary progesterone levels have been investigated to detect luteal deficiency. Other groups have looked at blood progesterone and salivary progesterone in carefully matched patients (age-matched but selected for breast symptoms or no breast symptoms, or breast cysts and no breast cysts) but nobody has managed to validate the difference that Mauvais Jarvis has shown.

The general feeling now is that the inadequate corpus luteum theory as an aetiological factor for benign breast disease is not valid. In fact if one looks at the whole range of possibilities of hormones, the whole field is very disappointing. A summary of many studies in a review by Wang and Fentiman reviewed the whole literature, and concluded that for progesterone the luteal deficiency theory is unproven [1]. Oestradiol has also been studied carefully, but no gross abnormality was shown, nor any abnormality that was reproducible between studies. More recently people have said that free oestradiol should be investigated but again some studies have come out showing no real differences. Despite the universally accepted theory that oestrogen must be implicated, it is very hard to prove.

There have been many studies on prolactin and an overall summary of them all is that if one looks at benign disease versus age-matched asymptomatic controls, no abnormality of basal prolactin can be shown.

There have been some interesting papers, including some from our own group, that have looked at a stimulation of prolactin release using thyrotropin releasing hormone (TRH), and there are now five or six studies with carefully matched patients that have demonstrated an increased peak release of prolactin to TRH. The mechanism of this is not known, but it can be demonstrated that patients with severe symptoms have a peak release of prolactin higher than controls. In Cardiff we have demonstrated that women with cyclical mastalgia have a higher peak prolactin than women with non-cyclical mastalgia. In addition the height of the peak prolactin response is a predictor of whether those women will respond to subsequent endocrine manipulation. Prolactin might therefore be interesting, but on random basal levels there are no differences.

There have been many studies on gonadotropins and androgens but it is very difficult to show abnormalities. This is not only in benign disease. People who have tried to show differences in breast cancer patients have also had many disappointments in trying to show differences between disease state and non-disease state when looking at hormones. Serum levels of hormones do not help us very much.

The incidence of breast pain in many British studies of women coming to a general practitioner (GP) is 50%. It is thus very very common. Much of it is minimal and does not cause disturbance to the lifestyle. But many of these patients are referred to the breast clinic. In the Cardiff breast clinic the proportion of patients coming with breast pain as the primary symptom for referral is 45%. Many of these patients the GP sees are then referred on for specialist opinion. Not all of these 45% need treatment. Many have come because they fear cancer, and when told that they do not have cancer then they are happy with that. Our own experience in Cardiff is that the proportion of patients who require treatment for mastalgia is only of the order of 8% of our new cases, and in fact we only evaluate that 8% and treat about 4%. Treatment of benign symptoms is therefore only needed in a small proportion.

The question is can this 4% of women with severe pain be helped. Many studies of bromocriptine, including a recent multicentre study in Europe just completed with more than 270 patients entered, randomized between bromocriptine and placebo, have confirmed that suppression of

161

prolactin will reduce breast symptoms. A study with danazol also showed that both breast pain and nodularity could be suppressed much better with the drug than with placebo.

The group at Guy's have performed studies showing a reduction of symptoms on tamoxifen, whether one uses 10 mg or 20 mg. The side-effects are higher on 20 mg. Other studies have shown that both evening primrose oil and low fat diets also reduce symptoms.

Cystic disease is a problem. The fear of malignancy due to the presentation of a lump is well known. It has been estimated that in western society some 7% of women will develop a macrocyst at some time which will need the attention of a doctor. Women who have multiple cysts will have to come back recurrently because they have a high rate of recurrent cyst formation. Cystic disease is therefore a problem for both the clinician and the patient. Clinical assessment of a nodular breast full of cysts is sometimes impossible, and radiologically it is not easy because of accompanying fibrosis.

It is worth attempting to treat women with multiple cysts. In Nottingham patients with multiple recurrent cysts were treated with danazol (300 mg/day) and a placebo treatment was used in the controls. This trial showed that the danazol-treated patients had fewer total new cysts over the period of follow up, by both clinical (aspirated), and radiological criteria. There was only a 38% cyst re-formation rate in the treated group compared with 91% in the controls. These data have been confirmed by many people, in that women with multiple recurrent cysts have a high likelihood of getting further cysts in the next year. There is further evidence from Scandinavia. Rasmussen *et al.* performed a similar study and also showed reduction in symptoms and a reduction of the number of aspirated cysts using danazol. A randomized trial is now in progress to determine whether Zoladex is effective in the treatment of breast pain. Clearly danazol has a major effect on reducing cyst formation but nobody is absolutely clear on how danazol works in this situation.

Can proliferative change in the breast be reduced? There is some circumstantial evidence. There are links between cystic disease and proliferation of the breast. Proliferative changes are very common in association with cystic disease. In danazol-treated patients with cystic disease there is a reduction in the density of mammograms, and this presumably is a reduction in the ductolobular units as well as a reduction in fibrosis. It is thought that danazol should not affect the fat content of the breast.

There is the well-known finding of reduction of benign breast disease, including cystic disease, in patients on long-term oral contraceptives. There is no hard evidence, it is all circumstantial. There are no current models to study this in animals. Studies are needed which show whether hormonal manipulation can affect proliferative changes

In Cardiff a large number of women who had cysts were compared with age-matched women who only had nodularity. Age-specific breast cancer incidence rates were calculated for these women and also woman years of follow up. Their cancer risk was also calculated. These patients have a follow up of at least 5 years up to a maximum of 12 years. Women who had multiple cysts aspirated had a higher risk of developing breast cancer. The histology of the patients in this study who had been biopsied was then examined. There were 27 patients who had only had nodularity and had never had a cyst aspirated, 19 who had had only one cyst aspirated, and 45 patients who had had multiple cysts aspirated. These patients subsequently, for other reasons, went on to have a biopsy and tissue was available. The incidence of apocrine change across the groups and epithelial hyperplasia was very interesting in that the multiple cyst group had significantly more mild and florid hyperplasia then the other two groups, and there was also one case of atypia in this group. This suggested that there was increased epithelial hyperplasia in association with cystic disease.

The rate of cancer development in this group of patients was also investigated. In patients who had apocrine change but no epithelial hyperplasia, the observed number of cancers was five and there was no significant difference with the non-biopsied population. However, cancers occurred in the epithelial hyperplasia patients in the hyperplastic groups, as one might expect from the data. Thus the patients with benign disease who go on to develop cancer are those who have the pathological marker of risk, namely hyperplasia.

REFERENCE

1. Wang, D.Y. and Fentiman, I.S. (1985). Epidemiology and endocrinology of benign breast disease. *Breast Cancer Res. Treat.*, **6**, 5–36

Discussion III

Dr Nicholson

We know that the pituitary gland is very important for both mammary gland development and for maintaining the growth of breast tumours. Mammary glands do not develop well in hypophysectomized animals and there have been suggestions from certain clinical trials that tamoxifen is not very effective in patients that have been hypophysectomized. So given that this is the situation, that having developed compounds that do not have great central activity might work against them being effective antitumour agents if that is an important mechanism in the growth of breast cancer?

Dr Wakeling

I agree. What I have presented today is what might be called the super-optimist's view. I am sure that others think that there are very good reasons why pure antagonists might not be as acceptable as a partial agonist.

Dr Howell

What effect will this drug have on ovarian function in premenopausal women when we give it to them, and what effect will it have on their bones?

Dr Wakeling

As far as ovarian function is concerned, I cannot give a definitive answer to that question. We have in progress at the moment a series of experiments in female monkeys in which we are actually measuring the uterus in terms of myometrial and endometrial volumes using nuclear magnetic resonance, and in those studies we are also looking at the ovaries. It is too early to give a definitive answer and I would not say anything one way or the other. As far as bones are concerned, we have done measurements in rats in the sort of study I have described where we have measured LH and weight and uterine weight and so on, and in those studies we have been unable to detect a significant loss of bone in the animals at drug doses which give effective involution of the uterus. Not only are we saying that there is a potency difference between peripheral and central targets of oestrogen action, but there are also – and this is really no surprise to anybody who knows the biology of steroids – very significant differences in the threshold of action of oestrogen at different peripheral target organs.

We do not understand why that is so, and that does not tell us anything about what might happen to bone density in women on pure antioestrogen treatment. Only that of course it has recently become evident that if anything tamoxifen has an oestrogenic effect on bone in women as it does indeed on bone in rats. In fact, tamoxifen is a potent oestrogen on bone in rats in terms of preventing bone loss in oophorectomized animals.

Professor Mansel

Professor Blamey did point out that the prognostic factors for conservation may well be different from the ones he presented. Would he give us some explanation why that should be? One would expect that say the intrinsic factors would also predict for local invasiveness or resistance to radiotherapy. What other factors are likely? Vascular invasion was mentioned.

Professor Blamey

On our analysis the factors which emerged as significant were vascular invasion and young age – and this is now also reported from all the French series. It is very unusual to see a local recurrence after conservation in a woman aged > 50; it is the 30-year-olds who are getting these local recurrences in the breast.

Vascular invasion within the tumour seems to be a very powerful factor, and that emerges in all the French analyses as well as our own.

Vascular invasion is probably reflecting the sort of tumour that is permeated fairly widely in the breast because it is often lymphatic invasion, and that may be one of the reasons. A combination of grade, surrounding DCIS and vascular invasion may explain why the young women are getting these recurrences in the breast.

Mr Preece

Professor Blamey has made a very cogent case for why we should adopt a prognostic index. The problem which most of us have had about using it is the one that he described, the fact that we do not have the pathologists. The move ahead, the ability now for this to be done as a relatively unskilled method will make the system more easily applicable in other places.

But how did he derive the utility codes which were part of the index?

Professor Blamey

By the Cox analysis, a multivariate analysis which gives two values. It gives the beta-value, which indicates the weight of the index, and the Z-value which is the relation of the beta-value to its standard error. That gives the fact of whether it is significant or not. The Cox analysis simply describes the cut-off level for significance for those factors.

Mr Preece

Say we in this room decided we would like to apply the index. Would it be necessary for us to derive our utility coefficients in our particular disease populations or could we take on board and expect to work those which have been derived in Nottingham?

Professor Blamey

Several other people have followed this index. Moneypenny applied it to Birmingham data. They had had a different method of lymph node biopsy so it was just applying the lymph node biopsy positive or negative and produced very good curves. Bennett applied it in Australia, where they did not have grading but used oestrogen receptor instead. They had a slightly more complicated index, but again it worked out very well. A group in Canada have seen the index, applied it to their data and again it has come up with very good curves. So every centre can design their own prognostic index according to which type of data they are recording.

Dr Klijn

What is the consequence diagnostically and therapeutically for the patients in whom tumour cells were found in their bone marrow?

Professor Eiermann

We already treat node-positive patients with adjuvant therapy and we are treating the node-negative patients with a positive marrow.

Dr Klijn

In a randomized study?

Professor Eiermann

It is a randomized study, together with another clinic. They have started on this programme too. We are treating with tamoxifen in the postmenopausal receptor-positive patients or with adjuvant chemotherapy in the other patients.

Dr Klijn

But there are no results?

Professor Eiermann

No data.

Mr Preece

Has it been possible to correlate the findings with any of the relatively new tumour markers?

Professor Eiermann

We have not done this. We are starting now to compare results with the epidermal growth factor receptor (EGF) and with other prognostic factors, ploidy and such things, but this work is still in progress.

Dr Klijn

Are there data on the incidence of the presence of the EGF receptor in bone marrow tumour cells?

Professor Eiermann

No. We could not demonstrate them – we published this 6 months ago. We could demonstrate immunological changes in the bone marrow in those patients who have micrometastasis or tumour cells. We could clearly show that there is a reduction in the interleukin receptor in this area in the bone marrow where we found the tumour cells, and some changes in the CD1:CD4 ratio can clearly be demonstrated. So we suppose that there might be a local event preceding the development of micrometastasis in the bone marrow.

Dr Klijn

Were the bone marrow aspirates taken during surgery for the primary breast cancer?

Professor Eiermann

Yes. We do the primary surgery and we have shown that it does not matter if we do the bone marrow puncture after surgery or before surgery. The patients do not suffer with this method. We have six puncture sites, which is a lot, but we have had no complications or problems in 5 years.

Mr Bundred

Does it really matter which of the two antibodies is used to stain presumed metastases when they are looked at at recurrence?

Professor Eiermann

We started with the anti-EMA antibody. Everybody knows about the discussion that took place in 1984–85 in several British journals. There is a false positive staining reaction of the anti-EMA antibody with plasma cells and we have recognized and analysed this problem. We have changed the antibodies. We used primarily the anti-EMA and the LICRLON, and in patients 40 to 100 we used cytokeratin antibody in addition. The panel of antibodies seems to enhance the staining intensity and seems to enhance the rate of detection. So now we are using a panel of antibodies. We are no longer using one antibody but three antibodies.

Professor Mansel

If there are several antibodies, is it one particular antibody that ticks the bad prognosis patients, or does it not correlate with any?

Professor Eiermann

It does not correlate.

Dr Klijn

What are you now planning to do in Dundee?

Mr Preece

On the national front in Scotland we have been working quite hard in the last 12 months on the successor to our tamoxifen trial, and I guess like everybody else we have recognized that we must accept the results of the various adjuvant Nolvadex trials in that virtually everybody, certainly the node-positive patients, must receive tamoxifen. And so our studies will be thinking about the question of what we can conveniently add which will be useful to improve the adjuvant results.

We are really still very much in debate on this. We have just sent round to all the surgeons in Scotland and all the radiotherapists and all the people who treat breast cancer a questionnaire offering them a number of options. But I do not think I am spilling any secrets if I report that one of the most popular ideas at the moment would be to try to use a regimen in which there is some form of perioperative perisurgical short-term addition to the adjuvant therapy.

Dr Klijn

A single treatment or a combination with long-term treatment?

Mr Preece

A combination. The new element over and above Nolvadex being the short-term perioperative modality.

R. Karesen

Just for clarity, are you now talking about Stage I cancers or are you talking about Nolvadex for everybody?

Mr Preece

The Scottish trial I have just discussed is concerned with the whole group of operable breast cancers. But from our own Scottish data we are encouraged to believe that we should continue to use Nolvadex in the global study.

There really are two areas in which trials can be conducted. There is the group of trials in which one hopes to bring in as many clinicians as possible who are treating patients but who perhaps do not have the facilities for using these sophisticated prognostic determinants such as tumour markers and the proteins, and so for that group, that is to say for the nationwide Scottish trial, we would be including the Stage I diseases and we would be providing a recipe there for blanket adjuvant Nolvadex in Stage I. But for the centres with the abilities to do these tests we will be looking in a more detailed way at whether we can see if indeed the pious hope which I have expressed in this talk, that we can actually select the bad-risk and the good-risk patients, enables us to choose at the start. There are so many of the delegates who are very involved in trials themselves. I wonder if I might just ask whether they in their own countries feel that our knowledge now about the effects of adjuvant therapy in Stage I disease is such that the time has come to mount really large studies using these prognostic discriminants. Does anybody have strong views about that?

Dr Klijn

In our centre at present we do not treat patients with node-negative tumours.

Mr Preece

Not even with adjuvant tamoxifen?

Dr Klijn

Not even that. But at present we are planning such trials based on the discrimination possible by the modern prognostic factors.

Mr Preece

As a corollary to that, in terms of the clinicians in Holland who allow their patients to be included in trials, what proportion of such clinicians would have the facilities for doing assays of the protein and so on?

Dr Klijn

The modern ones or the classical ones?

Mr Preece

Both really.

Dr Klijn

The classical ones are still receptor levels. All laboratories can do that examination and that is generally done throughout the Netherlands. But the number of patients entering trials is very low and they are mainly in the cancer centres in the university hospitals and some interested general hospitals. But overall the percentage of patients entering trials is very low and we have to stimulate that in the Netherlands.

Mr Preece

Only a very small proportion of all patients with breast cancer would have receptor assays done in Britain.

Dr Klijn

What about Scotland? What is the percentage of patients entering trials? Do they all go into trials?

Mr Preece

No. A very small proportion of the total.

Dr Klijn

What advice about treatment is given to the patients who are not included in trials when their nodes are negative, as a standard treatment. Are they put on tamoxifen, or nothing?

Mr Preece

The point about the large proportion of patients who do not go into trials is that they are patients who are not in my charge or my care and so I imagine they get a variety of different treatments. But because they do not go into trials, because the way they are treated is not recorded and published, we do not know what the generality of clinicians use. So I cannot answer the question because I do not know the answer.

Dr Klijn

We were told that plasma markers may be useful for discrimination between high and low risks and there was a mention of CA15-3. Do you have any experience with that?

Mr Preece

We have. This is within the University of Dundee rather than in the Scottish national context. We have now had the opportunity of studying quite a large series of patients with CA15-3 and the results suggest very strongly that it might well be a method of identifying patients who are likely to do badly from the outset.

Dr Klijn

At time of diagnosis of the primary tumour and what percentage of patients has increased levels?

Mr Preece

Yes, and of patients with clinically locoregional disease about 15%.

Dr Klijn

Your double-blind randomized study with Zoladex? After a month you will know which of the patients have had Zoladex and which have not, mainly based on the disappearance of menstruation.

Professor Mansel

It is a problem. There were similar problems with danazol. We have addressed this problem in several different ways. One is to not make a definite enquiry. The clinician who assesses the symptoms does not enquire of the patient; that is what we did in the danazol study. The clinician does not ask about menstruation and somebody else records the side-effects. Another way is to base the assessment on the patient's evaluation using linear analogues. But I accept the point. The problem is that where menstruation disappears obviously the change is mentioned. But then placebo-treated patients also have disappearance of menstruation. This is the interesting thing. If we look at the placebo studies, many many times a proportion of the patients will have similar side-effects to the treated group. It may seem as though it is easy for the patients to say whether or not they are on the treatment but in practice that is not so.

Dr Klijn

How many patients have now been treated?

Professor Mansel

One hundred and seventy, half with Zoladex and half not. It is a 50% randomization.

Mr Preece

As one of the participants in that study I shared the apprehension which existed about sham injections, and I would reinforce absolutely that it has not been a problem with the patients.

The point that Dr Klijn raised has not been such a problem as I anticipated and in addition to the amenorrhoea from sham injections, it is also extraordinary how many other side-effects have developed and been reported in patients who have sham injections. I know the results are not available yet, but in our own cohort of 20 patients in this group it is quite remarkable. In a sense, being involved for the very first time in a study with a sham injection, I am impressed by the strength of the placebo effect and suggest that it is something to take note of.

At the end of his presentation Professor Mansel put out a tantalizing aperitif. He says he is deriving a study in which he is hoping there will be a marker for epithelial hyperplasia. Would it be fair for us to hear more about what this might be?

Professor Mansel

That is a good question and we have had problems with that. What we are currently measuring or working on is EGF. We are also not only trying to get a measure on hyperplasia but activity within the breast. We shall also be looking at Hagenson's cyst fluid protein. I accept that that does not tell us of hyperplasia within the hyperplastic parts of the section, but as we all know there is no marker of hyperplasia. We are still not certain. We are leaving it open. We shall take the specimens and try probably a number of monoclonal antibodies and look and see which one might give us a measure.

Obviously the ideal way would be to either have a circulating marker, which would be marvellous, or failing that to do a biopsy. But of course ethically it is very difficult when one has treated a patient with cystic disease and got rid of the cystic disease to then ask to biopsy her breast. Some people have done these studies. I do not know how they managed to do it. There are other ways we can do it. We could take a fine needle aspiration and look at a cytological effect. We can look at markers of hormone activity within cytological preparations, and we shall do that if we can.

The answer is we do not have a certain marker and we shall have to make deductions whether there has been an effect or not. The important or interesting point about all this is if one can reduce the hyperplasia where does that leave the long-term cancer risk. This is the same question as tamoxifen treatment for prophylaxis.

Dr Colin

Has Zoladex been used in gross cystic disease?

Professor Mansel

Have I used it? No. That is my next trial. I am committed to this trial now but I think it is an interesting concept. We will have the data from the study I have just shown in symptoms in the breast, not cystic disease but symptoms. I have data on that and I have data from bromocriptine-treated patients and data from danazol-treated patients, so I shall be able to make some comparisons.

I would expect that if Zoladex does reduce breast symptoms in the study just shown, then based on the effect that danazol has on symptoms in cysts, one would assume that Zoladex would help breast cysts.

But we do not know the mechanism of macroscopic breast cystic disease. Nobody knows why those tiny cysts, which we know many women have, become macrocysts. The switch from one to the other is unclear. We firmly believe that macroscopic cystic disease is a different disease from the woman who has a random histological biopsy and it shows microcystic disease. That is nothing. That is normality. We do not believe that multiple recurrent macrocysts is normality. We believe it is abnormality.

Professor Eiermann

Has there been any attempt to combine Zoladex with progesterone so as to relieve the symptoms of Zoladex injection?

Professor Mansel

I have not thought about it. We have not yet done the formal analysis and so I am not certain what our level of side-effects is likely to be in premenopausal women with benign disease.

R. Karesen

Professor Mansel mentioned the interesting paper from Page and DuPont showing an increased risk ratio if a patient has hyperplasia. I am not sure I understood it correctly, but he suggested that if such patients were given danazol, or perhaps Nolvadex, that risk might be reduced. Does he put patients on those preparations and is there any evidence from the literature that it will really help in risk reduction.

Professor Mansel

As I said, it is all speculative. I have no hard evidence that that is so. I am making a deduction that if a patient has cysts in the breast, as we showed in our material and others have shown very commonly she will also have epithelial hyperplasia somewhere in that breast. Not in the cyst necessarily, maybe in a ductolobular tissue to one side of the cyst. If the cyst is reduced, and we can measure that, whether by aspiration, ultrasound or whatever, what has happened to the accompanying hyperplasia? The answer is I do not know. What I am putting forward is speculative and I have no data to make that point. But if we could do that then it would be a very interesting possibility. Of course we would have to bear in mind all the other problems of long-term treatment and of side-effects.

But as I said at the start the several trials I have now done show that if breast symptoms are suppressed with a short course of endocrine therapy they remain suppressed when the endocrine therapy is taken away.

I am very intrigued at why a short course of endocrine therapy has a prolonged effect on the breast. If we think about conventional steroid actions we would say that that is not really possible, because once the hormones are back, the turnover of the receptor is quite fast and things should go back to normal. But they do not go back to normal. And so something very interesting is happening. One could postulate treating high-risk patients say, not continuously for life but for short bursts. We would treat for 3 months, leave for a year and treat again for 3 months. Maybe we could do it this way. But I do not know. These are just thoughts on the subject.

R. Karesen

To be a touch provocative. What do you do in Cardiff if the pathologist says there is a hyperplasia, or there is atypia? Do you put them on tamoxifen?

Professor Mansel

I would first go and see my pathologist and find out what he means by hyperplasia. If it is hyperplasia with atypia, which we know is only 4% of biopsies, I just watch the patient and do not put her on tamoxifen. I do not yet believe the evidence is strong enough to do that – for the reasons already discussed, that we do not know that we can reduce the hyperplasia.

Dr Klijn

My own experience is with six patients treated with LHRH agonist depot preparation for 6 months. In all the six patients the symptoms disappeared completely or disappeared significantly. They were all women with severe mastalgia. But at the end of the treatment, the symptoms recurred in the majority, although not to the same level in all of them. With respect to the aetiology there are some reports showing high levels for growth factors in cystic fluids.

Professor Mansel

There is a lot of information on cyst fluids and many things are extreme in them. DHA sulphate is an example and Miller has done a lot of work on this. The problem has been trying to correlate that biochemical finding with an event in the breast, either recurrence or cyst size, cyst volume, colour of fluid. None of these correlate very well. The only thing that seems to correlate is the two populations based on ion concentration. But unfortunately our experience of that has been we agree that the two populations can be split, but in our hands it has not been very predictive of the behaviour of subsequent cyst formation. The Edinburgh group says it is, and they also claim it is predictive, or it may be predictive, of breast cancer risk. They have not produced the data for that because they are currently trying to recall these patients and get these data, but they hope to have them out very soon. We are doing a similar study to see whether we can show that it is a cancer risk predictor, but I cannot say that it is at the moment.

Index